Microdosing Magic

Unveiling the Transformative Power of Psychedelic Mushrooms

By True Eira

Ancient Wisdom for Modern Healing

Visit

trueeira.com/test

Find Your Microdose Personality

TRUE
EIRA

ABOUT AUTHOR

"Microdosing Magic: Unveiling the Transformative Power of Psychedelic Mushrooms" is a collective masterpiece spearheaded by Travis Eric and the True Eira team. Travis, an adept mushroom cultivator, brings a grassroots-level expertise to the practice of microdosing, particularly in its application for personal growth and mental clarity.

The True Eira team, with diverse backgrounds, adds depth, combining scientific study with practical application. Their exploration extends beyond traditional uses, offering nuanced insights into the psychological and spiritual benefits of microdosing. This book is a culmination of their extensive research and experience, providing a comprehensive guide that transcends conventional understanding, aimed at those seeking to enhance their lives through mindful and informed use of microdosing.

TRUE
EIRA

Disclaimer: The information provided in this book is for general informational purposes only. The author makes no representations or warranties of any kind, express or implied, about the completeness, accuracy, reliability, suitability, or availability of the information contained in this book. Any reliance you place on such information is strictly at your own risk.

Table of Contents

Visit

trueeira.com/test

Find Your Microdose Personality

TRUE
EIRA

Introduction

In recent years, a quiet revolution has been brewing in mental health, personal growth, and wellness. As the stigma surrounding psychedelics dissolves slowly, a burgeoning interest in their therapeutic potential has emerged. Among these powerful substances, microdosing psychedelic mushrooms has captured the attention and curiosity of people from all walks of life. "Microdosing Magic: Unveiling the Transformative Power of Psychedelic Mushrooms" aims to provide a comprehensive and accessible guide to understanding the practice of microdosing and how it can enhance various aspects of our lives.

The renaissance of psychedelic research has brought forth a wealth of knowledge, revealing the multifaceted benefits and potential risks of microdosing. Focusing on sub-perceptual doses of psilocybin-containing mushrooms, this book delves into the science, history, and practical applications of microdosing, offering a roadmap for those seeking to explore this transformative practice responsibly and intentionally.

As you embark on this journey, you'll discover how microdosing can unlock creativity, enhance focus, improve athletic performance, foster emotional well-being, and deepen your connection to yourself and the world around you.

With expert guidance and real-life examples, "Microdosing Magic" aims to illuminate the potential of psychedelic mushrooms as a tool for personal growth, self-discovery, and healing, ultimately empowering you to harness their transformative power for a more fulfilling, enriched, and balanced life.

The Renaissance of Psychedelic Research

In the last few decades, we have witnessed a resurgence of interest in psychedelic substances, particularly in mental health and wellness. Many factors, including a growing dissatisfaction with conventional treatments for mental health disorders, new scientific techniques, and a cultural shift towards holistic approaches to well-being, have fueled this renaissance of psychedelic research.

In the early 1990s, the seeds of the modern psychedelic renaissance were sown as several dedicated and forward-thinking researchers set out on a mission to unlock the therapeutic potential of psychedelic substances, including LSD, MDMA, and psilocybin—the active compound found in psychedelic mushrooms. This exciting wave of research emerged due to loosening restrictions on psychedelic investigations, which had been tightly regulated since the 1960s due to political and social concerns about the possible risks associated with their recreational use.

As the restrictions eased, these pioneering researchers were able to delve deeper into the potential benefits of psychedelics, uncovering their potential to transform mental health treatment and enhance personal development. Along the way, they discovered the unique properties of psilocybin and its ability to promote healing, self-discovery, and connection to the world around us. Numerous studies and anecdotal evidence suggest that psychedelics may offer promising solutions to some of society's most pressing mental health challenges.

The resurgence of interest in psychedelic research has also inspired a new generation of scientists and therapists to further explore these substances' potential for healing and personal growth. Today, clinical trials and studies reveal promising results for treating various mental health disorders, including anxiety, depression, PTSD, and addiction. As more people become aware of the potential benefits of psychedelics, the stigma surrounding their use is slowly dissipating, making way for a future where these powerful substances can be utilized responsibly and effectively to improve our collective well-being.

One of the most significant developments has been the growing body of evidence supporting the use of psychedelics in treating mental health disorders. Early studies, conducted primarily in the 1990s and 2000s, showcased promising results for treating anxiety, depression, and PTSD. These foundational investigations paved the way for more recent studies that have honed in on psilocybin, especially for its potential to alleviate treatment-resistant depression, anxiety related to terminal illness, and addiction. The remarkable outcomes of these studies have fueled a renewed interest in the healing potential of psychedelics, inspiring researchers and mental health professionals to explore their potential further.

Another key factor driving the resurgence of interest in psychedelics has been the emergence of cutting-edge neuroimaging techniques, such as functional magnetic resonance imaging (fMRI) and magnetoencephalography (MEG). These advanced tools have granted researchers unprecedented access to the brain's inner workings, allowing them to delve deeper into how psychedelic substances interact with our neural networks. As a result, researchers have been able to shed light on the underlying mechanisms that may contribute to the therapeutic effects of psychedelics, unlocking new possibilities for understanding and harnessing their healing potential.

With the combination of groundbreaking research and innovative neuroimaging techniques, the field of psychedelic therapy has evolved rapidly in recent years, promising to transform how we approach mental health treatment. The growing acceptance of psychedelic substances as legitimate therapeutic tools is a testament to the tireless efforts of researchers, mental health professionals, and advocates who have challenged long-held misconceptions and stigma. As we continue to learn more about the transformative power of psychedelics, we stand on the brink of a new era in mental health care that embraces the full potential of these remarkable substances to heal, inspire, and connect to the world around us.

The growing body of evidence supporting the therapeutic potential of psychedelics has been accompanied by a cultural shift towards more holistic and integrative approaches to mental health and well-being. As our understanding of the complex interplay between the mind, body, and spirit deepens, there has been a renewed interest in the role that altered states of consciousness, such as those induced by psychedelics, can play in promoting psychological healing and personal growth.

Within this broader context of the psychedelic renaissance, microdosing has emerged as a popular and increasingly well-researched approach to harnessing the potential benefits of psychedelic substances. By taking small, sub-perceptual doses of these compounds, individuals can experience subtle shifts in perception, mood, and cognition without the intense, immersive experiences typically associated with full-dose psychedelic trips.

As we explore the history, science, and potential benefits of microdosing psychedelic mushrooms in the following chapters, we hope to contribute to a growing dialogue about these powerful substances' responsible and intentional use as tools for transformation and healing.

The Concept of Microdosing

Microdosing involves taking tiny amounts of psychedelic substances, like psilocybin, from magic mushrooms, LSD, or other entheogens. The goal is to experience slight improvements in cognitive function, creativity, and emotional well-being without a full psychedelic trip's powerful, reality-shifting effects. A sub-perceptual dose is usually around one-tenth to one-twentieth of a standard recreational dose, depending on the substance used.

The primary objective of microdosing is to promote positive changes in daily life without experiencing the potentially overwhelming effects associated with higher doses. Those who practice microdosing frequently report enhancements in mental clarity, mood, creativity, focus, problem-solving abilities, and an increased sense of connection to the world around them. Many individuals choose to incorporate microdosing into a holistic approach to self-improvement, mental health, and personal growth, ultimately transforming their lives in meaningful ways.

The concept of microdosing can be traced back to the early days of psychedelic research when scientists and therapists began experimenting with low doses of substances like LSD to comprehend their effects on the human brain better. One of the trailblazers in this field was Dr. Albert Hofmann, the Swiss chemist who first synthesized LSD in 1938. In his later years, Hofmann advocated for microdosing, describing it as a method to access the potential benefits of psychedelics without experiencing the intense hallucinogenic effects that may hinder day-to-day functioning.

As microdosing has evolved, it has garnered significant attention from researchers, mental health professionals, and individuals seeking alternative pathways to self-improvement and well-being. By integrating microdosing into various aspects of their lives, people have found innovative ways to tap into the transformative potential of psychedelics while maintaining a balanced and grounded lifestyle. The growing interest in microdosing is a testament to the resilience of the human spirit and our collective desire to explore new avenues for personal growth, healing, and connection with the world around us.

While microdosing has gained popularity in recent years, it is not a new phenomenon. Many indigenous cultures have a long history of using plant medicines, such as the Amazonian brew ayahuasca, in low doses for various purposes, including healing, divination, and enhanced cognitive function. In Western culture, the concept gained mainstream attention with the publication of Dr. James Fadiman's book "The Psychedelic Explorer's Guide" in 2011. Fadiman's work provided practical guidelines for microdosing and helped to legitimize the practice in the eyes of the public.

Today, microdosing is the subject of growing scientific interest as researchers explore its potential benefits and risks. While the available evidence is still limited, early studies suggest that microdosing may have a range of therapeutic applications, from addressing mental health disorders such as depression and anxiety to enhancing creativity and cognitive function in healthy individuals. As our understanding of the science behind microdosing continues to evolve, this practice will likely play an increasingly important role in the emerging field of psychedelic medicine and wellness.

Purpose of the Book

The primary purpose of this book is to provide a comprehensive, evidence-based, and accessible guide to microdosing psychedelic mushrooms. As interest in microdosing continues to grow and the renaissance of psychedelic research flourishes, there is a pressing need for reliable information on the topic grounded in scientific understanding and practical experience. This book aims to fill that gap by offering a balanced and nuanced exploration of the potential benefits, risks, and applications of microdosing and practical guidance on incorporating this practice into one's life responsibly and intentionally.

The book is designed to serve a diverse audience, from individuals curious about microdosing and its potential benefits to mental health professionals, researchers, and policymakers interested in the evolving landscape of psychedelic medicine. Through scientific research, personal anecdotes, and practical advice, we seek to empower readers with the knowledge and tools they need to make informed decisions about microdosing and engage with this practice to support their personal growth, mental health, and overall well-being.

In addition to providing an in-depth exploration of the science, history, and practicalities of microdosing psychedelic mushrooms, the book also aims to contribute to a broader dialogue about the responsible and ethical use of psychedelic substances in our society. As we continue to learn more about the potential of these mighty compounds to promote healing, enhance creativity, and deepen our connection to ourselves and the world around us, we must engage in open, honest, and evidence-based discussions about how to integrate these substances into our lives in a way that honors their transformative potential while minimizing risks.

Ultimately, this book aims to catalyze personal and societal transformation by providing a roadmap for those curious about the possibility of microdosing psychedelic mushrooms to improve their mental health, enhance their creativity, and support their journey of self-discovery and growth. By fostering a deeper understanding of this practice and its potential applications, we hope to contribute to the ongoing renaissance of psychedelic research and to help shape a future in which these powerful substances are recognized and valued for their transformative potential.

Understanding Psychedelic Mushrooms

Delving into the fascinating world of psychedelic mushrooms uncovers a rich tapestry of history, culture, and many potential benefits. As we explore the realm of these enigmatic fungi, it's crucial to understand their origins, the compounds responsible for their effects, and the different types of mushrooms that fall under the psychedelic umbrella.

Since ancient times, psychedelic mushrooms have significantly influenced diverse cultures' spiritual and healing practices worldwide. They have captivated the minds of scholars, artists, and adventurers alike, inspiring a sense of awe and reverence for their seemingly mystical properties. As modern science delves deeper into the complex mechanisms behind their effects, we are beginning to unravel the secrets hidden within these fungi and gain a deeper appreciation for their potential applications in medicine and personal growth.

Tracing the history and cultural significance of psychedelic mushrooms, we learn about the primary types of mushrooms that contain psychoactive compounds and delve into the chemistry of psilocybin and psilocin, the active ingredients responsible for their effects. As we explore the intricate world of these remarkable organisms, we gain the essential knowledge needed to navigate the transformative practice of microdosing.

History and Cultural Significance

Psychedelic mushrooms, also known as "magic mushrooms," have a long and fascinating history that spans various cultures and continents. The use of these mushrooms, which contain the psychoactive compounds psilocybin and psilocin, dates back thousands of years and is deeply interwoven with diverse societies' spiritual and healing practices.

The earliest evidence of the use of psychedelic mushrooms can be traced back to prehistoric times, as indicated by rock paintings and other artifacts discovered in regions such as North Africa, Mesoamerica, and Europe. In the Mesoamerican cultures, particularly the Aztecs and the Mazatecs, the use of magic mushrooms was an integral part of their religious rituals, serving as a means to communicate with the divine, seek guidance, and facilitate healing.

In the 16th century, the Spanish conquest of the Americas led to the suppression of indigenous spiritual practices, including the use of magic mushrooms. However, the use of these mushrooms persisted in secret, particularly among the Mazatec people in the mountains of Oaxaca, Mexico. It was in the mid-20th century that the Western world became aware of the existence and properties of magic mushrooms, primarily due to the work of ethnomycologist R. Gordon Wasson.

Wasson's groundbreaking 1957 article in Life magazine, which documented his experiences with magic mushrooms during a Mazatec ceremony led by the shaman Maria Sabina, introduced the Western world to the psychoactive effects of psilocybin and sparked a surge of interest in the potential therapeutic and spiritual applications of these substances.

In the 1960s, researchers such as Timothy Leary and Richard Alpert (later known as Ram Dass) began exploring the psychological and spiritual effects of psychedelic substances, including psilocybin, LSD, and mescaline. This period saw a rapid increase in the recreational use of psychedelics and the emergence of the counterculture movement, which embraced these substances as tools for personal growth, creativity, and social change.

However, the widespread recreational psychedelic use during this time led to backlash and criminalization of these substances in the late 1960s and early 1970s. This backlash marked the beginning of a decades-long period of strict regulation and limited research into the potential benefits of psychedelics, which persisted until the early 1990s.

As we have seen in recent years, the renaissance of psychedelic research has brought renewed attention to the potential therapeutic and transformative properties of magic mushrooms and other psychedelic substances. Within this context, microdosing has emerged as a popular and increasingly well-researched approach to harnessing the benefits of these compounds in a more subtle and controlled manner.

Throughout history and across cultures, magic mushrooms have held a unique place in the human experience as powerful tools for spiritual exploration, healing, and self-discovery. As we continue to learn more about the potential of these remarkable fungi, we must approach their use with the respect, intentionality, and curiosity they deserve, honoring their rich cultural heritage while exploring new ways to integrate their transformative potential into our modern lives.

Main Types of Psychedelic Mushrooms

There are over 180 species of mushrooms that contain the psychoactive compounds psilocybin and psilocin, which are responsible for inducing the characteristic psychedelic effects. While each species may have unique properties and potency, several psychedelic mushrooms stand out as the most commonly known and used. This section will provide an overview of the main types of psychedelic mushrooms.

Psilocybe cubensis

Psilocybe cubensis includes a variety of popular strains such as "Golden Teacher," "Mexicana," "B+," and "Penis Envy," or is simply referred to more generally as "cubes." It is one of the most popular and widely cultivated psychedelic mushrooms. It is native to regions of Central and South America, Southeast Asia, and the Gulf Coast of the United States. P. cubensis is relatively easy to cultivate and has moderate potency, making it a popular choice for beginners and experienced users.

Psilocybe semilanceata

Psilocybe semilanceata, commonly known as "Liberty Caps," is a widely distributed species native to Europe, North America, Asia, South America, and parts of Oceania. It is characterized by its small size and distinctive conical cap shape. Liberty Caps are considered to be moderately potent and are often sought after by foragers due to their prevalence in the wild.

Psilocybe azurescens

Psilocybe azurescens, or "Flying Saucers," is a highly potent species of psychedelic mushrooms native to the Pacific Northwest region of the United States. It is known for its strong visual effects and intense spiritual experiences. Due to its high potency, P. azurescens is often recommended for experienced users seeking a more powerful psychedelic experience.

Psilocybe cyanescens

Psilocybe cyanescens, also known as "Wavy Caps," is another highly potent species native to the Pacific Northwest region of the United States and parts of Europe. This species is easily recognizable when bruised by its wavy cap edges and strong bluing reaction. P. cyanescens is sought for its intense visual effects and profound spiritual experiences.

Psilocybe tampanensis

Psilocybe tampanensis is a rare species of psychedelic mushrooms found initially in Florida, United States, and later in Mississippi. This species is known for producing "magic truffles" or "Philosopher's Stones," which are the sclerotia (underground compact masses of mycelium) containing psilocybin and psilocin. P. tampanensis has a moderate potency and is often used for microdosing due to its milder effects than other species.

Panaeolus Cyanescens

Panaeolus cyanescens, commonly called the "Pans," is a potent species of psychedelic mushrooms native to various regions worldwide, including Central and South America, Australia, and parts of North America. This species is known for its distinctive jet-black spore print and the blue bruising reaction when the mushroom's tissue is damaged, hinting at its high psilocybin content. It prefers to grow in dung or well-manured ground and is often found in pastures or other grassy areas. P. cyanescens is known for its strong visual hallucinogenic effects and profound spiritual experiences, making it a popular choice among experienced users seeking a potent psychedelic journey.

These are just a few of the many species of psychedelic mushrooms found around the world. Each species has unique properties, potency, and effects. It is essential for individuals considering microdosing to carefully research and choose the appropriate type of mushroom for their needs and experience level. In addition, it is crucial to ensure proper identification and sourcing to avoid consuming toxic or dangerous mushrooms.

The Active Compounds: Psilocybin and Psilocin

Psychedelic mushrooms owe their mind-altering effects to the presence of two primary active compounds: psilocybin and psilocin. Both of these compounds are tryptamines, structurally similar to the neurotransmitter serotonin. They interact with serotonin receptors in the brain, particularly the 5-HT2A receptor, leading to the characteristic changes in perception, cognition, and emotion associated with psychedelic experiences.

Psilocybin (4-phosphoryloxy-N,N-dimethyltryptamine) is magic mushrooms' most abundant psychoactive compound. It is a prodrug, meaning it is biologically inactive until metabolized. When ingested, psilocybin is rapidly dephosphorylated by alkaline phosphatase enzymes in the liver and converted into psilocin (4-hydroxy-N,N-dimethyltryptamine), which is the compound responsible for the majority of the psychedelic effects.

Psilocin is structurally similar to serotonin (5-hydroxytryptamine) and the powerful psychedelic compound DMT (N,N-dimethyltryptamine). It is more lipid-soluble than psilocybin, allowing it to readily cross the blood-brain barrier and interact with serotonin receptors in the central nervous system.

Psilocin's affinity for the 5-HT2A receptor is believed to be the primary driver of the psychedelic effects. However, it also binds to other serotonin receptor subtypes, which may contribute to the overall experience.

The intensity and duration of the psychedelic experience depend on various factors, including the dose, the individual's metabolism, and the specific mushroom species. The effects of psilocybin and psilocin usually begin within 30 to 60 minutes of ingestion and can last anywhere from 4 to 8 hours, with peak effects typically occurring between 1.5 to 3 hours after ingestion.

When microdosing psychedelic mushrooms, the goal is to consume a sub-perceptual dose of psilocybin and psilocin, typically about one-tenth to one-twentieth of a full recreational amount. The compounds are believed to produce subtle changes in perception, mood, and cognition at these low doses without causing the intense visual, auditory, and sensory distortions of a full psychedelic experience. The growing interest in microdosing has sparked a surge of research into the potential therapeutic applications of these compounds, with early studies suggesting that they may offer a range of benefits, from alleviating depression and anxiety to enhancing creativity and cognitive function.

The Science of Microdosing

Microdosing has gained considerable attention in recent years, with many people seeking to harness the potential benefits of psychedelic substances without the intensity of a full-blown psychedelic experience. By taking small, sub-perceptual doses, individuals aim to enhance various aspects of their lives, from creativity and focus to emotional well-being and personal growth. But what exactly is the science behind microdosing, and how does it work on the brain?

As we venture into microdosing, it's essential to understand the underlying principles that make this practice so intriguing and potentially transformative. Researchers are hard at work exploring the effects of microdosing on the brain, uncovering the mechanisms through which these subtle doses may bring about significant changes in cognition, mood, and perception. By investigating the potential benefits and risks associated with microdosing, we can begin to paint a clearer picture of this innovative approach to self-improvement and healing.

In this journey, we will define what microdosing entails and examine the current state of scientific research on the topic. We will delve into how microdosing can impact the brain and discuss the potential benefits and risks associated with this practice. As we uncover the science of microdosing, we will equip ourselves with the knowledge to make informed decisions about whether and how to incorporate microdosing into our lives for optimal well-being and growth.

Defining Microdosing

Microdosing is consuming small, sub-perceptual doses of psychedelic substances, such as psilocybin-containing mushrooms, LSD, or other entheogens, to achieve subtle enhancements in cognitive function, creativity, and emotional well-being without experiencing the intense, reality-altering effects typically associated with a full psychedelic trip. A sub-perceptual dose is approximately one-tenth to one-twentieth of a typical recreational dose.

The objective of microdosing is to facilitate positive changes in day-to-day life without the potentially overwhelming effects of a higher dose. Individuals who engage in microdosing often report improvements in mental clarity, mood, creativity, focus, problem-solving abilities, and a greater sense of connection to the world around them. Many people who practice microdosing do so as part of a holistic approach to self-improvement, mental health, emotional health, and personal growth.

The concept of microdosing has gained significant attention in recent years, thanks in part to the work of researchers and authors such as Dr. James Fadiman, who has provided practical guidelines for microdosing and helped to legitimize the practice in the eyes of the public. However, the scientific literature on microdosing is still relatively limited, and much of the existing knowledge on the topic is derived from anecdotal reports, case studies, and preliminary research.

Early studies have suggested that microdosing may hold promise as a therapeutic intervention for a range of mental health conditions, including depression, anxiety, and PTSD, as well as a tool for enhancing cognitive function, creativity, and overall well-being in healthy individuals. The mechanisms underlying these effects are not yet fully understood, but they are thought to involve a combination of changes in brain activity, neuroplasticity, and neurotransmitter levels, particularly serotonin.

Despite the growing interest in microdosing and its potential benefits, many questions still need to be answered. As the science of microdosing continues to evolve, researchers, clinicians, and individuals who engage in this practice must approach it with curiosity, open-mindedness, and a commitment to rigorous scientific inquiry.

The Effects of Microdosing on the Brain

While research on the effects of microdosing is still in its early stages, preliminary studies and anecdotal reports suggest that the practice can have a range of subtle yet potentially significant impacts on brain function. This section will provide an overview of the current understanding of the neural mechanisms underlying the effects of microdosing on cognition, mood, and perception.

Neuroplasticity and neurogenesis: One of the most promising areas of research on microdosing involves its potential to promote neuroplasticity and neurogenesis, which are the brain's ability to adapt, rewire, and create new neural connections in response to new experiences and information. Psychedelic compounds like psilocybin and psilocin have been shown to increase the expression of brain-derived neurotrophic factor (BDNF), a protein that supports neuron growth, survival, and differentiation. This increase in BDNF may contribute to enhanced learning, memory, and cognitive flexibility in individuals who practice microdosing.

Serotonin receptor activation: As mentioned earlier, psilocybin and psilocin are structurally similar to the neurotransmitter serotonin and interact primarily with the 5-HT2A receptor in the brain. This receptor involves various cognitive and emotional processes, including mood regulation, perception, and learning. Activation of the 5-HT2A receptor by psilocin is thought to play a vital role in the subjective effects of microdosing, such as improved mood, reduced anxiety, and increased creativity.

Changes in brain connectivity: Studies on the effects of full-dose psychedelic experiences have shown that these compounds can induce profound changes in brain connectivity, leading to increased communication between regions that do not typically interact. While the effects of microdosing on brain connectivity have not been extensively studied, the practice could lead to more subtle shifts in neural communication patterns, contributing to enhanced cognitive function, creativity, and problem-solving abilities.

Modulation of the default mode network: The default mode network (DMN) is a network of interconnected brain regions active when the mind is at rest and not focused on the outside world. The DMN has been implicated in self-referential thinking, rumination, and mind-wandering. Research on full-dose psychedelic experiences has shown that these compounds can reduce the activity and connectivity within the DMN, leading to a dissolution of the sense of self and a decrease in rumination. While the effects of microdosing on the DMN are not yet well understood, the practice could lead to subtle changes in DMN activity, which could contribute to improved emotional well-being and reduced symptoms of depression and anxiety.

It is important to note that research on the effects of microdosing on the brain is still in its infancy, and many questions remain unanswered. As the field continues to grow, it will be essential for researchers to conduct rigorous, well-designed studies to elucidate further the neural mechanisms underlying the effects of microdosing and to determine the safety, efficacy, and long-term consequences of this practice.

Potential Benefits and Risks

As microdosing gains popularity, there has been a growing interest in understanding its potential benefits and risks. While research on microdosing is still in its early stages, preliminary studies and anecdotal reports suggest that the practice may offer a range of benefits for mental health, cognitive function, and overall well-being. However, it is also essential to consider the potential risks and drawbacks associated with microdosing.

Potential Benefits:

<u>Improved mood and emotional well-being</u>: Many individuals who engage in microdosing report experiencing improvements in mood, reduced anxiety, and increased overall emotional well-being. Preliminary research has supported these claims, with some studies showing promising results in treating depression, anxiety, and PTSD.

<u>Enhanced cognitive function</u>: Microdosing has been associated with increased focus, creativity, and problem-solving abilities, as well as better mental clarity and a heightened capacity for learning. These cognitive enhancements may benefit individuals in creative or intellectually demanding fields.

<u>Increased energy and motivation</u>: Anecdotal reports suggest that microdosing can lead to increased energy levels, greater motivation, and improved productivity, which could have a positive impact on both personal and professional pursuits.

<u>Heightened self-awareness and personal growth</u>: Microdosing may facilitate greater self-awareness, emotional intelligence, and introspection, promoting personal growth and self-improvement.

Potential Risks:

<u>Legal and regulatory issues</u>: Using psychedelic substances, including psilocybin-containing mushrooms, is illegal in many jurisdictions. Microdosing may expose individuals to legal and regulatory risks, depending on their location.

<u>Adverse psychological effects</u>: While many individuals report positive experiences with microdosing, some may experience

adverse psychological effects, such as increased anxiety, paranoia, or emotional instability. It is essential for individuals considering microdosing to be aware of their personal mental health history and any potential risk factors.

Lack of standardized dosing and quality control: As microdosing is not regulated, there is a risk of inaccurate dosing and variability in the potency and quality of the substances being used. This lack of standardization could lead to unintended effects or negative interactions with other medications or substances.

Unknown long-term effects: The long-term effects of microdosing are not yet well understood, and there is a lack of research on the potential risks associated with chronic, low-dose exposure to psychedelic substances.

In summary, microdosing may offer a range of potential benefits for mental health, cognitive function, and overall well-being. Still, it is important to approach the practice with caution and awareness of the potential risks and drawbacks. Further research is needed to understand better the safety, efficacy, and long-term consequences of microdosing. Individuals considering this practice should carefully weigh the potential benefits against the risks and consult a healthcare professional if necessary.

Sourcing and Identifying Psychedelic Mushrooms

Sourcing and identifying psychedelic mushrooms is an important aspect of microdosing for those who engage in this practice. Accurate identification is crucial to ensure safety and avoid accidental ingestion of toxic species. This section provides an overview of common psychedelic mushroom species, tips for identification, and responsible sourcing practices.

Common psychedelic mushroom species: There are over 180 species of mushrooms that contain the psychoactive compounds psilocybin and psilocin. Some of the most common species include:

- Psilocybe cubensis: This species is one of the most popular and widely available due to its ease of cultivation and moderate potency.
- Psilocybe semilanceata: Commonly referred to as "Liberty Caps," these mushrooms are known for their distinctive shape and are typically found in grassy, damp areas across North America and Europe.
- Psilocybe cyanescens: Known as "Wavy Caps," these mushrooms are characterized by their wavy caps and bluish coloration when bruised. They are native to the Pacific Northwest and parts of Europe.

Tips for identification: Proper identification of psychedelic mushrooms is essential for safety. While it is beyond the scope of this section to provide a comprehensive guide to mushroom identification, some general tips include:

- Consult reliable field guides and online resources for accurate descriptions, photographs, and habitat information.
- Learn about the distinctive features of psychedelic mushrooms, such as cap shape, gill color, spore print color, and bruising reaction.
- Become familiar with toxic lookalike species that can cause harm if ingested.
- Connect with experienced foragers or mycologists in your area to help with identification and to learn about local species.
- Always exercise caution and verify the identity of any mushroom you intend to consume.

Responsible sourcing practices: There are several responsible and ethical ways to source psychedelic mushrooms, including:

- Foraging: If you have the knowledge and experience to identify psychedelic mushrooms, foraging in the wild safely can be a sustainable and rewarding option. Be sure to follow local regulations, respect private property, and practice ethical foraging by leaving some mushrooms behind to allow for spore dispersal and future growth.
- Cultivation: Growing your own mushrooms from spores or mycelium can provide a reliable and controlled source of psychedelic mushrooms. Be aware of the legal implications of cultivating psychedelic mushrooms, as it may be illegal in some jurisdictions.
- Purchasing: In some countries and regions where psychedelic mushrooms are legal or decriminalized, they can be purchased from reputable sources. Always verify the identity and potency of purchased mushrooms, and ensure they are sourced ethically and sustainably.

It is important to note that the possession, cultivation, and consumption of psychedelic mushrooms may be illegal in some jurisdictions. Always be aware of and comply with local laws and regulations.

Sourcing and identifying psychedelic mushrooms is a critical aspect of engaging in microdosing. Accurate identification is essential for safety, and responsible sourcing practices ensure sustainability and ethical consumption. By taking the time to learn about common species, identification tips, and responsible sourcing, individuals can better navigate the world of psychedelic mushrooms and engage in microdosing with greater confidence and care.

Creating a Microdosing Schedule

Developing a well-structured microdosing schedule is a critical component of a safe and effective microdosing experience. Adhering to a schedule can help minimize potential side effects, prevent tolerance build-up, and create opportunities for proper integration and reflection. In this section, we will discuss the importance of a microdosing schedule, highlight popular scheduling protocols, and offer tips for personalizing your schedule.

A microdosing schedule is crucial for several reasons. Firstly, adhering to a schedule can help manage the frequency and intensity of potential side effects, ensuring a safer and more comfortable experience. Secondly, taking regular breaks between microdosing sessions can help prevent tolerance development, allowing for consistent effects and long-term benefits. Lastly, a well-planned schedule provides dedicated time for integrating insights and reflecting on how microdosing impacts personal growth and well-being. By incorporating these considerations into a carefully crafted plan, individuals can optimize their microdosing experience and maximize its positive effects.

Popular Microdosing Protocols

Before beginning a microdosing regimen, there are a few aspects to consider. Firstly, many newcomers to microdosing often report feelings of sleepiness or fatigue. If you experience fatigue during the initial months of your microdosing journey, it is likely a sign that the mushroom medicine is aiding in the relaxation and balance of your nervous system. For example, if your lifestyle has been characterized by a rapid pace, overworking, excessive intake of stimulants, and insufficient rest, the microdoses might prompt sleepiness to promote recovery. If you encounter this feeling, it's recommended that you allow yourself to rest. This tiredness should diminish once you've adequately restored your energy.

Secondly, some individuals experience experience slight headaches when they first start microdosing. This is typically seen as a mild detoxification response. The mushrooms are thought to help heal the nervous system and in certain instances, trigger neural repair. To enable this, the removal of specific toxins from the brain might be needed, which can lead to headaches. If you encounter this, it's suggested that you drink plenty of purified water and proceed at a pace that feels right for you. This side effect usually subsides after approximately a week.

The strain of mushrooms you choose for microdosing can significantly influence your experience. Most commonly, people microdose with Psilocybin cubensis. However, expert mushroom breeders have been meticulously selecting and cross-breeding various cubensis strains from diverse locations, isolating different phenotypes from these strains based on their preferred characteristics. These unique strains can sometimes have vastly different effects at both microdose and macro dose levels.

For instance, the 'Golden Teachers' strain tends to instill clarity and confidence in users at microdose levels. 'Jack Frosts' can help you tap into your compassion and elicit a sensation akin to meditating or performing yoga for an hour. The 'Mexicana' strain generally helps users to feel more relaxed. 'Stormtroopers' are known to boost energy and can assist you in completing more reps at the gym. 'Phobos' can provide comfort, enveloping you like a warm, feel-good blanket.

In contrast, 'Albino Penis Envy', often abbreviated as 'APEs', may induce restlessness or anxiety. Therefore, it's crucial to identify the strain you're microdosing with and observe the differences. This will help you pinpoint the strains that best suit your needs and preferences under various circumstances.

Select a microdosing protocol that aligns with your needs and preferences. It's important to restate that the effects of mushrooms can become less consistent when taken consecutively over several days. Therefore, scheduling days of rest between doses is advisable, allowing your tolerance levels to recalibrate. Above all, the key is to experiment and familiarize yourself with how the mushrooms interact with your body. This process will help you determine an appropriate dosage and frequency that suits your comfort level and complements your lifestyle.

Here are a few examples of commonly followed protocols:

The Fadiman Protocol: Named after Dr. James Fadiman, is a well-known and widely used microdosing regimen. This protocol advocates taking a microdose of a psychedelic substance on Day 1, followed by two days of abstinence (Days 2 and 3), and then resuming microdosing on Day 4. This cycle is repeated, with microdoses taken once every three days.

The rationale behind this schedule is to ensure that the body and mind have ample time to rest and integrate the effects of each microdose. By allowing for a two-day break between doses, individuals can avoid building a tolerance to the substance and minimize the risk of potential side effects. Furthermore, this schedule enables users to observe and assess the impact of microdosing on their mental, emotional, and physical well-being over an extended period.

Adhering to the Fadiman Protocol can help individuals maximize the potential benefits of microdosing while minimizing risks. This approach provides a structured and balanced microdosing regimen that can be safely incorporated into one's daily routine, fostering personal growth and well-being in a controlled and manageable manner.

The Stamets Stack: Designed by the esteemed mycologist Paul Stamets, it is an alternative microdosing schedule emphasizing a more frequent dosing pattern. In this protocol, individuals take a microdose every day for five consecutive days, followed by a two-day break. The purpose of the two-day hiatus is to avert tolerance buildup and provide an opportunity for integration of the microdosing experience.

The daily microdosing in the Stamets Stack can lead to more consistent exposure to the substance, potentially providing more stable and ongoing benefits for individuals with PTSD. However, it is essential to monitor one's response to this protocol closely, as the increased frequency of dosing may not be suitable for everyone. By following the Stamets Stack, users can explore a different microdosing approach that may be more effective for their particular needs and circumstances while ensuring a structured and safe regimen.

Paul Stamets, in addition to recommending the specific dosing schedule for the Stamets Stack, also advises incorporating certain natural supplements to enhance the overall benefits of the microdosing experience. The combination of substances he proposes is often called the "Stamets Stack."

Stamets suggests combining the psilocybin microdose with two other supplements: lion's mane mushroom (Hericium erinaceus) and niacin (vitamin B3). Lion's mane mushroom is believed to support cognitive function, neurogenesis, and overall brain health. Niacin is a vasodilator, which helps increase blood flow and circulation in the body, potentially aiding in the distribution and efficacy of the psilocybin and lion's mane.

The idea behind this synergistic combination is that each substance contributes to the enhancement of cognitive function and the promotion of neuroplasticity, working together to optimize the overall benefits of the microdosing experience. By including lion's mane and niacin, the Stamets Stack aims to create a more comprehensive and effective approach to microdosing for individuals seeking cognitive and mental health benefits, including those with PTSD.

The 1-1-1 Protocol: The 1-1-1 Protocol, which consists of alternating microdosing days with rest days, allows individuals to experience the potential benefits of microdosing more consistently throughout the week while offering an opportunity for integration and preventing excessive exposure to the substance. This microdosing pattern can help individuals maintain a balanced state of mind, as the effects of the microdose may carry over into the rest day. Many people enjoy the off-days more than the days they microdose, noticing residual positive effects which some describe as an "afterglow."

By following the 1-1-1 Protocol, individuals may find it easier to observe the subtle effects of microdosing on their mood, cognitive function, and overall well-being, as they have a shorter interval between doses. This can be particularly useful for those seeking relief from PTSD symptoms, as the more frequent dosing schedule may provide sustained support for emotional regulation and resilience.

Additionally, the 1-1-1 Protocol allows for greater flexibility and can be adjusted based on personal preferences or individual responses to microdosing. For example, if someone finds the effects too intense or experiences unwanted side effects, they can easily modify the protocol by extending the rest period or reducing the microdose amount.

The Balanced Protocol: The Balanced Protocol offers a unique approach to microdosing that combines the benefits of more frequent dosing with sufficient rest periods to promote optimal results. By microdosing on Days 1-4, individuals can experience the potential positive effects of magic mushrooms on mood, cognition, and PTSD symptoms more consistently while still allowing their system to reset during the three-day break.

This dosing pattern can be particularly beneficial for those who want to maintain a steady routine and reap the potential advantages of microdosing throughout the workweek, with weekends reserved for rest and integration. The three-day break also helps to minimize the risk of developing a tolerance to the substance, ensuring that the microdoses remain effective over time.

The Balanced Protocol can be customized based on individual needs and preferences. For instance, if someone finds that four consecutive days of microdosing is too intense, they can adjust the protocol to include an additional rest day in between or decrease the microdose amount.

Travis Eric's Protocol: The Travis Eric Protocol is an unconventional approach to microdosing that emphasizes "filling up" the body with mushrooms by taking microdoses more frequently throughout the day and week. This protocol involves microdosing 5-7 days a week and taking doses in the morning, sometimes dosing again in the afternoon, and occasionally at night. As tolerance builds, the dosage is increased slightly to accommodate the body's adaptation to the substance.

With this approach, the effects of microdosing will still be noticeable but will become less predictable overall. However, after a month or two, individuals might notice a decreased desire for microdosing altogether. At this point, it's essential to listen to the body and take a break for a couple of weeks or more. After the "filling up" period, the need for microdosing may further diminish, and one might feel more sensitive to taking microdoses, leading individuals to dose only once or twice a week or less.

Dosing this way can allow a person to build a deeper relationship with the mushrooms. The mushrooms will work more on the individual's awareness, enhance their emotional body, tune them into their feelings, and have an increased heart-opening effect.

The Travis Eric Protocol presents a unique, more intensive microdosing method for those interested in exploring its potential advantages in greater depth. This protocol could be seen as an 'emotional warrior' path and may not be suitable for everyone.

Before embarking, it is recommended to establish a balanced foundation in your life. This includes developing a solid understanding of mindfulness, maintaining a consistent meditation practice, adhering to a healthy diet, and incorporating regular physical exercise into your routine.

However, as this approach involves a more frequent dosing schedule, it's essential to be mindful of the associated risks. Careful monitoring of one's reactions and responses to this regimen is a critical aspect of ensuring safety and effectiveness. It's also important to only use this protocol for a maximum of 2-3 months before taking a long break.

Customized schedules: Some individuals may prefer to develop a personalized schedule based on their unique needs, symptoms, and response to microdosing. You might microdose on specific days of the week, such as Monday, Wednesday, and Friday, or adjust the frequency and duration based on your experiences and progress.

Pay attention to any emotional experiences that may arise, new sensitivities you might encounter, and the heightened awareness you may develop about yourself and others. As the mushrooms work to harmonize and heal your heart and mind, you'll likely become more attuned to your inner self and the world around you.

As with any microdosing protocol, consulting a healthcare professional or an experienced guide is highly recommended. Prioritize self-care and listen to your body and mind throughout the microdosing journey to ensure a safe and beneficial experience.

Remember that microdosing is a highly individualized process, and it may take some trial and error to find the most effective protocol and schedule for you. Be patient, track your experiences, and make adjustments as to optimize your microdosing journey

Personalizing your Microdosing Schedule

Creating an optimal microdosing schedule may vary between individuals due to personal goals, sensitivity to psilocybin, and lifestyle. To establish a personalized schedule that suits your unique needs, consider the following steps:

Start by choosing a popular protocol: Select one of the well-known microdosing protocols as a foundation, using it as a guideline for your journey. This can provide a reliable starting point from which you can fine-tune your schedule according to your experiences and personal requirements.

Keep a detailed journal: Documenting your microdosing experiences is vital for understanding its effects on your well-being. Record information such as dosage, timing, and the impact of each microdose. Be sure to note any side effects, emotional shifts, or insights gained throughout the microdosing process. This will help you track your progress and make any necessary adjustments to your schedule.

Reflect on your experiences and adjust as needed: Periodically review your journal entries to assess your overall microdosing experience. Reflect on the patterns and trends you notice and consider whether your current schedule aligns with your personal goals. Make adjustments to your schedule, dosage, or frequency of microdosing as needed, based on your observations and objectives.

Listen to your body and mind: Paying close attention to your body's signals and reactions to microdosing is crucial for a successful experience. Be mindful of any changes in your physical, emotional, and mental states, and adjust your schedule or dosage accordingly. This will help you minimize side effects and maximize the benefits of microdosing.

Incorporate mindfulness practices: Enhance the benefits of microdosing by incorporating mindfulness practices, such as meditation, yoga, or breathwork, into your routine. These practices can help you deepen your self-awareness and support the integration of insights and personal growth facilitated by microdosing.

Seek support and guidance: Connecting with others who have experience with microdosing or consulting with a professional can provide valuable insights and support. Sharing your experiences and learning from others can help you optimize your microdosing journey and maximize its positive impact on your life.

By following a well-structured microdosing schedule and tailoring it to your needs, you can minimize side effects, prevent tolerance, and allocate time for integration and reflection. This personalized approach will help ensure a successful and beneficial microdosing experience that supports your overall well-being and personal growth.

Accurate Dosing and Measurement

Ensuring accurate dosing and measurement is a crucial aspect of microdosing with psychedelic mushrooms. Proper dosing helps minimize potential side effects, maximize potential benefits, and create a consistent and controlled experience. This section covers the importance of accurate dosing, different methods of measurement, and tips for determining an appropriate microdose.

Importance of accurate dosing: Accurate dosing is essential for a safe and effective microdosing experience. Inaccurate dosing can lead to several issues:

- Unintended effects: Taking too much may result in a more intense experience than desired, which could cause anxiety, paranoia, or other adverse side effects.
- Inconsistent results: Inaccurate dosing can lead to variable outcomes, making it difficult to determine the effectiveness of microdosing for personal growth and well-being.
- Tolerance development: Overdosing may lead to the development of tolerance, requiring higher doses for the same effects and potentially diminishing the long-term benefits of microdosing.

Methods of measurement: There are several methods for measuring an accurate dose of psychedelic mushrooms:

- Digital scale: A digital scale with a resolution of at least 0.01 grams is recommended for precise measurement. Weigh the dried mushrooms to determine the desired dose.
- Volumetric dosing: This method involves dissolving a known quantity of ground mushrooms in a measured volume of liquid (such as water or alcohol). The solution is then divided into equal parts to create consistent doses. This method can help account for variations in potency between different parts of the mushroom or different mushrooms within the same batch.
- Capsules: Grinding dried mushrooms into a fine powder and filling capsules with a measured amount of the powder can provide a consistent and convenient dosing

method. Capsule machines are available to make this process easier.

Determining an appropriate microdose: Individual responses to microdosing can vary, and finding the right dose for your needs and goals is essential. A general guideline for a microdose of psilocybin-containing mushrooms is 1/10th to 1/20th of a typical recreational dose. For Psilocybe cubensis, this usually equates to approximately 0.1 to 0.3 grams of dried mushrooms.

To find your optimal dose, start with a lower amount (e.g., 0.1 grams) and gradually increase the dose in small increments over several microdosing sessions until you find the right balance of effects and minimal side effects. It's also possible to take a .1 gram microdose, and if the feeling is not sufficient after 40 minutes to 1 hour, supplement with an additional .1 gram to increase the effect. The effect will build on itself in a diminishing way as tolerance develops, which is why it's important to take breaks to maintain a consistent feeling.

Different mushrooms have different potency, start small and increase the dose small until you find what works for you. Follow a microdosing schedule, such as one day on, two days off, or every fourth day, to prevent the development of tolerance and maintain the effectiveness of microdosing. Keep a journal to track changes in your mood and behavior over time. Results can be subtle but profound and will build on themselves over time. The days you microdose will be good days. Still, the mushrooms also work on your mind and emotional body over time, allowing you to experience more subtle effects like increased emotional sensations and an opening of the heart.

Accurate dosing and measurement are critical aspects of microdosing with psychedelic mushrooms. By ensuring proper dosing, individuals can minimize potential side effects, maximize benefits, and create a consistent and controlled microdosing experience. Using reliable measurement methods and carefully determining an appropriate dose can help individuals engage in microdosing safely and maintain a more predictable experience.

Setting and Intention

Embarking on any journey of self-exploration or personal growth demands mindfulness and intentionality. The practice of microdosing psychedelic mushrooms is no exception. The importance of setting and intention cannot be overstated when engaging in such a transformative experience. These two critical components not only serve as guiding principles for navigating the microdosing process but also help to maximize its potential benefits while minimizing any risks or undesirable outcomes.

Setting refers to the physical and emotional environment in which the microdosing takes place, while intention encompasses the personal goals, motivations, and mindset that drive the individual's decision to microdose. By carefully cultivating a supportive setting and clarifying one's intentions, the individual can create a strong foundation for a successful and meaningful microdosing journey.

In this exploration, we will discuss the significance of setting and intention in the context of microdosing, offering practical guidance on how to create a nurturing environment and cultivate a clear and purposeful mindset. We will also delve into the role of intention in shaping the microdosing experience and provide insights on aligning your goals with your inner values and aspirations. As we uncover the importance of setting and intention, we will learn to approach microdosing with mindfulness and a deeper sense of purpose, ultimately enriching our journey toward personal growth and self-discovery.

Importance of Setting

The importance of setting in the context of microdosing psychedelic mushrooms cannot be overstated. Setting refers to the physical, emotional, and social environment in which microdosing occurs. It plays a crucial role in shaping the individual's experience and can significantly influence the outcomes and potential benefits of microdosing.

A supportive and comfortable setting can greatly enhance the microdosing experience by providing a safe space for self-exploration and personal growth. When individuals feel relaxed and secure in their environment, they are more likely to remain open to the subtle effects of microdosing and to better integrate the insights gained during the process.

Several factors contribute to creating an ideal setting for microdosing:

Physical environment: Ensure the space is clean, comfortable, and free from distractions. Natural light, plants, and pleasant scents can help create a calming atmosphere.

Emotional atmosphere: Cultivate a positive mindset and eliminate sources of stress or anxiety as much as possible. This may involve practicing relaxation techniques, such as deep breathing or meditation, prior to microdosing.

Social context: Surround yourself with supportive and understanding people, if possible. Engaging with like-minded individuals or participating in a microdosing community can provide valuable emotional support and encouragement during the process.

Timing: Choose a time when you can dedicate several hours to the microdosing experience without the pressure of work or other obligations. This will allow you to fully immerse yourself in the process and to reflect on your experience without feeling rushed.

By paying close attention to the setting, individuals can maximize the benefits of microdosing, minimize potential risks, and create a foundation for a successful and transformative journey.

Creating a Supportive Environment

A nurturing and comfortable space can help you remain open to the subtle effects of microdosing and better integrate the insights gained during the process. Here are some steps to create a supportive environment for your microdosing journey:

Choose a suitable location: Select a space that feels safe, comfortable, and private, where you can relax and focus on your experience. This could be a room in your home, a peaceful outdoor spot, or any other location where you feel at ease.

Personalize your space: Decorate the area with objects or elements that have personal meaning or evoke a sense of calm and serenity. This could include artwork, photographs, candles, or even your favorite blanket or cushion.

Minimize distractions: Eliminate potential interruptions by turning off electronic devices or informing those around you that you need some uninterrupted time for self-exploration and reflection.

Incorporate calming elements: Introduce soothing elements, such as soft lighting, calming scents, or gentle background music, to help create a peaceful atmosphere.

Prepare mentally: Engage in relaxation techniques, such as deep breathing, meditation, or mindfulness practices, to clear your mind and cultivate a positive mental state before microdosing.

Set clear intentions: Reflect on your motivations for microdosing and establish clear intentions for your journey. This can help guide your experience and provide a sense of direction and purpose.

Create a support network: Connect with like-minded individuals or participate in a microdosing community to share experiences, and insights and provide mutual support during your microdosing journey.

Schedule your microdosing sessions: Choose a time when you can dedicate several hours to the microdosing experience without the pressure of work or other obligations. This will allow you to fully immerse yourself in the process and reflect on your experience without feeling rushed.

Keep a journal: Document your thoughts, feelings, and insights during your microdosing journey to track your progress and facilitate self-reflection.

Be patient and open-minded: Remember that microdosing is a personal journey, and the effects may vary from person to person. Approach the experience with patience and an open mind, allowing yourself to explore and learn from the process.

Following these steps, you can create a supportive environment that fosters personal growth, self-exploration, and a positive microdosing experience.

Clarifying Intentions

Clarifying intentions is an essential step in the microdosing journey, as it helps you define the goals and purpose of your experience. By setting clear intentions, you can create a more focused and meaningful journey, paving the way for personal growth and self-discovery. Here are some tips to help you clarify your intentions for microdosing psychedelic mushrooms:

Reflect on your motivations: Consider why you are interested in microdosing and what you hope to achieve. This could be to enhance creativity, improve mental well-being, promote personal growth, or explore spiritual aspects of life.

Write down your intentions: Putting your intentions into words can help solidify your thoughts and make your goals more tangible. Keep a journal or a dedicated document to record your intentions and revisit them throughout your microdosing journey.

Be specific, yet flexible: While it's essential to have a clear idea of what you want to achieve, it's also important to remain open to unexpected insights and experiences. Recognize that your intentions may evolve and adapt as you progress.

Prioritize self-discovery: Focus on intentions encouraging self-exploration, personal growth, and self-improvement. This will help ensure that your microdosing experience is transformative and enriching.

Use visualization techniques: Visualize yourself achieving your intended goals or experiencing the desired benefits. This can help reinforce your intentions and make them feel more achievable.

Incorporate mindfulness practices: Engage in meditation, deep breathing, or other mindfulness exercises to cultivate a greater sense of self-awareness and presence. This will help you stay attuned to your intentions and maintain a deeper connection with your microdosing experience.

Revisit and reassess your intentions regularly: As you progress through your microdosing journey, take the time to reflect on your intentions and assess whether they still align with your goals and experiences. Adjust your intentions as needed to ensure they remain relevant and meaningful.

Share your intentions with a support network: Discussing your intentions with like-minded individuals or a trusted friend can provide valuable feedback, encouragement, and accountability throughout your microdosing journey.

By clarifying your intentions and regularly reflecting on them, you can create a more focused and purposeful microdosing experience, ultimately enhancing the potential benefits and personal growth derived from the process.

Diet and Lifestyle

Embarking on a microdosing journey with psychedelic mushrooms is an opportunity to not only explore your inner world but also to examine and optimize your overall well-being. Diet and lifestyle play a significant role in supporting the positive effects of microdosing and can enhance the transformative power of this practice. We will discuss the importance of a balanced diet, exercise, self-care, and other lifestyle factors that can help you maximize the benefits of your microdosing experience and improve your overall quality of life. By adopting a holistic approach, you can create a strong foundation for personal growth, emotional resilience, and lasting change.

Diet and Microdosing

Diet plays a crucial role in supporting the positive effects of microdosing with psychedelic mushrooms. A well-balanced and nutritious diet can help optimize your physical and mental well-being, allowing you to fully benefit from the microdosing experience. Here are some dietary considerations to keep in mind when microdosing:

Focus on organic whole foods: A diet rich in whole, unprocessed foods such as fruits, vegetables, organic whole grains, proteins, and healthy fats provides the essential nutrients your body and mind need to function optimally. These foods can support mental clarity, mood stability, and overall health during your microdosing journey. GMOs and Pesticides like glyphosate can contribute to gut dysbiosis, causing inflammation and even contributing to feelings of anxiety.

Stay hydrated: Adequate hydration is essential for maintaining cognitive function, energy levels, and overall well-being. Make sure to drink enough clean fluoride-free water throughout the day, especially when microdosing, as it may help to minimize potential side effects such as headaches or dizziness.

Limit caffeine and alcohol: Excessive caffeine consumption can exacerbate anxiety and interfere with sleep, while alcohol can negatively impact mood and cognitive function. Reducing or avoiding these substances during your microdosing journey can help you maintain a more balanced mental state and enhance the benefits of microdosing.

Choose serotonin-boosting foods: Foods rich in tryptophan, an amino acid that helps produce serotonin, can support a positive mood and emotional well-being. Examples of tryptophan-rich foods include turkey, chicken, fish, eggs, nuts, seeds, and legumes.

Opt for anti-inflammatory foods: Inflammation is increasingly linked to mental health issues such as depression and anxiety. Consuming anti-inflammatory foods, such as leafy greens, berries, fatty fish, nuts, and olive oil, can help support your mental well-being during your microdosing journey.

Eliminate Inflammatory Foods: Consuming a diet high in inflammatory foods can negatively impact both physical and mental health. Reducing or eliminating inflammatory foods from your diet may enhance the benefits of microdosing by promoting a healthier body and mind. Some common inflammatory foods to avoid or minimize include: Processed and refined sugars, trans fats (found in fried foods, processed snacks, and baked goods), Refined carbohydrates (white bread, pasta, and rice), Alcohol, Artificial additives and preservatives (Basically anything marketed and sold by the major food brands passed off as edible with an ingredient list you don't understand), Vegetable oils high in omega-6 fatty acids (such as soybean, canola, corn, and sunflower oils).

Maintain stable blood sugar levels: Eating regular meals and snacks, and focusing on complex carbohydrates, protein, and healthy fats, can help maintain stable blood sugar levels. This can reduce mood swings and irritability, supporting a more balanced emotional state during microdosing.

Pay attention to food sensitivities: Some individuals may have sensitivities to certain foods that can exacerbate mental health issues. If you suspect a food sensitivity, consider eliminating the potential trigger food from your diet and observe any changes in your mood or well-being. Notice how you feel when you eat grains, dairy, beans, or nightshades. Experiment with different diets until you find one that fits your body best.

Supplement wisely: While a well-balanced diet should provide most of the nutrients you need, certain supplements may be helpful in supporting your microdosing journey. Various supplements have been suggested to enhance the microdosing experience and support overall well-being. Some of these include:

1. Lion's Mane: This mushroom is known for its neuroprotective and cognitive-enhancing properties. It may boost memory, focus, and mental clarity, which could synergize with the effects of microdosing.

2. Niacin (Vitamin B3): Niacin has been suggested to improve circulation, support brain function, and assist with detoxification processes. Some people believe that niacin can enhance the effects of microdosing by increasing the availability of the psychedelic compound in the body.

3. L-Tyrosine: This amino acid is a precursor to neurotransmitters like dopamine, norepinephrine, and epinephrine. Supplementing with L-Tyrosine may help

support mood and cognitive function during microdosing.

4. Magnesium: Magnesium is an essential mineral that supports hundreds of enzymatic processes in the body, including those related to mood regulation and stress response. Supplementing with magnesium may help alleviate anxiety and promote relaxation during microdosing. Magnesium L-Threonate for the mind, magnesium malate for the daytime, and magnesium glycinate for the night.

5. 5-HTP: 5-Hydroxytryptophan (5-HTP) is a precursor to the neurotransmitter serotonin. Supplementing with 5-HTP may help support serotonin levels and promote a positive mood during microdosing.

6. Omega-3 Fatty Acids: These essential fats are known for their anti-inflammatory and neuroprotective properties. Consuming omega-3 supplements may support brain health and cognitive function during microdosing.

7. Rhodiola Rosea: This adaptogenic herb has been used to reduce stress, fight fatigue, and improve mental performance. Rhodiola may complement the effects of microdosing by supporting stress resilience and mental clarity.

8. Ashwagandha: Another adaptogenic herb, ashwagandha is known for its stress-reducing, anti-anxiety, and neuroprotective properties. It may help balance mood and support emotional well-being during microdosing.

9. B Vitamins: B vitamins are essential for maintaining optimal brain function and mental health. A B-complex supplement can provide a balanced source of these

essential nutrients, supporting overall well-being during microdosing.

10. Ginkgo Biloba: This herbal supplement has been used to improve memory, concentration, and blood flow to the brain. It may help enhance cognitive function and focus during microdosing.

11. Ubiquinol: This powerful antioxidant is the active form of Coenzyme Q10 (CoQ10) and plays a crucial role in cellular energy production and overall health. Ubiquinol supports mitochondrial function, which is essential for maintaining optimal brain function and energy levels.

It is important to note that not all supplements may be suitable for everyone, and individual responses may vary. Consult with a healthcare professional before adding any new supplements to your regimen, especially when microdosing with psychedelic mushrooms.

By paying attention to your diet and making conscious choices, you can support your body and mind during your microdosing journey, enhancing the overall experience and maximizing its potential benefits.

Exercise and Microdosing

Exercise and Microdosing: Combining physical activity with microdosing psychedelic mushrooms can potentially enhance the overall benefits of both practices. Exercise is known to improve mood, boost cognitive function, and increase overall well-being. When paired with microdosing, these effects may be amplified, leading to a more profound and transformative experience. Some potential synergies between exercise and microdosing include:

Enhanced focus and motivation: Microdosing can help increase focus and motivation, which may contribute to more effective and enjoyable workouts. By sharpening mental clarity and boosting energy levels, individuals may find it easier to engage in physical activity and maintain a consistent exercise routine.

Improved mind-body connection: Microdosing can heighten the mind-body connection, leading to increased self-awareness and better attunement to physical sensations. This heightened awareness may improve exercise form and technique, promote greater bodily control, and reduce the risk of injury.

Boosted mood and reduced stress: Both exercise and microdosing have been shown to help alleviate stress and improve mood. When combined, these practices may offer a synergistic effect, further enhancing emotional well-being and resilience.

Accelerated recovery: Microdosing may aid in reducing inflammation and promoting recovery after exercise, allowing for faster healing and reduced muscle soreness.

Expanded creativity: Microdosing is known to promote divergent thinking and creativity, which can be applied to exercise routines, inspiring new and innovative ways to stay active and engaged.

It's important to note that everyone's experience with microdosing and exercise may vary, and it is essential to start slowly and listen to your body's signals. Always consult a healthcare professional before combining microdosing with any new exercise routines or practices to ensure safety and optimal results.

Lifestyle Factors Influencing Microdosing Experiences

Lifestyle factors can significantly impact the effectiveness and experience of microdosing psychedelic mushrooms. By being aware of these factors and making necessary adjustments, individuals can maximize the benefits and minimize potential risks associated with microdosing. Some key lifestyle factors that can influence microdosing experiences include:

Sleep: Adequate and quality sleep is essential for overall well-being and cognitive function. Poor sleep can negatively affect mood, focus, and emotional stability, which in turn can impact the microdosing experience. Prioritizing a consistent sleep schedule and practicing good sleep hygiene can help create a solid foundation for microdosing.

Diet: Consuming a balanced and nutritious diet can support mental and physical health, enhancing the benefits of microdosing. Reducing or eliminating inflammatory foods, incorporating nutrient-dense whole foods, and staying hydrated can all contribute to a more positive microdosing experience.

Stress management: High stress levels can interfere with the effectiveness of microdosing, potentially exacerbating anxiety or emotional instability. Implementing stress-reduction techniques such as mindfulness meditation, yoga, or deep breathing exercises can help create a more conducive environment for microdosing.

Exercise: As mentioned earlier, regular physical activity can complement microdosing by enhancing focus, mood, and overall well-being. Engaging in consistent exercise can help amplify the benefits of microdosing and support a healthier lifestyle.

Setting and intention: The environment and mindset in which one approaches microdosing can significantly impact the experience. Creating a supportive and comfortable setting and clarifying one's intentions can help foster more positive and transformative experiences.

Social support: Building a network of supportive individuals who understand and respect the microdosing journey can be beneficial. Sharing experiences, discussing challenges, and seeking guidance from like-minded individuals can help foster a sense of community and support.

Self-monitoring and reflection: Keeping track of microdosing experiences, including dosage, frequency, and any effects, can help individuals tailor their approach and identify patterns. Regular self-reflection and introspection can also help integrate insights and lessons gained from microdosing into daily life.

By considering these lifestyle factors and making appropriate adjustments, individuals can create an environment that supports and enhances their microdosing experience, leading to more profound and lasting benefits.

Microdosing for Creativity and Cognitive Enhancement

In today's fast-paced and ever-evolving world, the quest for enhanced creativity and cognitive function has become more crucial than ever. Individuals across various fields—artists, entrepreneurs, scientists, and beyond—seek innovative ways to unlock their full potential and gain an edge in their personal and professional lives. Microdosing psychedelic mushrooms has emerged as a promising and increasingly popular tool for amplifying creative thinking and cognitive abilities.

This chapter delves into the fascinating world of microdosing for creativity and cognitive enhancement. We will explore the underlying mechanisms behind these benefits and discuss the ways in which microdosing can help improve problem-solving abilities, lateral thinking, and mindfulness. Drawing on case studies and personal anecdotes, we will shed light on the transformative potential of microdosing in unleashing the creative genius within.

Whether you are a seasoned creator searching for inspiration, a busy professional looking to enhance your mental clarity, or simply someone seeking new ways to expand your cognitive horizons, this chapter will provide valuable insights and practical guidance on how microdosing psychedelic mushrooms can elevate your creative and cognitive abilities to new heights.

Improving Problem-solving and Lateral Thinking

The practice of microdosing has gained popularity among individuals seeking to enhance their creativity, problem-solving skills, and cognitive function. By consuming small, sub-perceptual doses of psychedelic substances like psilocybin-containing mushrooms, users aim to achieve subtle improvements in mental clarity, focus, and innovative thinking without the intense, reality-altering effects of a full psychedelic experience.

Enhancing creativity: Many anecdotal reports and preliminary research suggest that microdosing can lead to increased creativity and divergent thinking, which are essential components of the creative process. Inducing subtle shifts in perception and cognitive flexibility, microdosing allows users to approach problems from new angles, make novel connections between seemingly unrelated concepts, and generate innovative ideas more effectively.

The exact mechanisms underlying these effects are not yet fully understood, but they may involve the activation of serotonin receptors, changes in brain connectivity, and increased neuroplasticity, as previously discussed. These neural changes could facilitate a more open, flexible, and expansive state of mind, creating an environment conducive to creative thinking and exploration.

Improving problem-solving and lateral thinking: Lateral thinking, or the ability to solve problems using indirect, creative approaches, is another cognitive skill that may be enhanced by microdosing. By promoting a more flexible and open-minded mental state, microdosing could help users overcome cognitive biases, identify alternative solutions, and think "outside the box" more effectively.

In addition to promoting lateral thinking, microdosing may also improve general problem-solving abilities by increasing mental clarity, focus, and the ability to make connections between seemingly unrelated information. These cognitive enhancements are particularly valuable in complex, intellectually demanding tasks that require innovative thinking and adaptability.

Balancing creativity and functionality: One of the key advantages of microdosing for creativity and cognitive enhancement is its potential to provide subtle, manageable effects that do not interfere with daily functioning. While a full psychedelic experience can be profoundly transformative, it may also be overwhelming and disorienting, making it challenging to integrate the insights gained during the experience into everyday life.

Microdosing, on the other hand, allows users to harness the potential cognitive benefits of psychedelic substances in a controlled, focused manner, striking a balance between creative exploration and practical functionality. This balance is particularly appealing to individuals working in creative fields or those seeking to enhance their problem-solving and lateral thinking abilities in professional or personal contexts.

In conclusion, microdosing holds promise as a tool for enhancing creativity, problem-solving, and lateral thinking. However, more research is needed to fully understand the underlying mechanisms and potential risks associated with this practice.

Enhancing Mindfulness and Focus

Microdosing has gained attention not only for its potential to boost creativity and problem-solving abilities but also for its ability to enhance mindfulness and focus. Many individuals who engage in microdosing report increased concentration, mental clarity, and a heightened sense of presence in their day-to-day lives.

Cultivating mindfulness: Mindfulness is the practice of maintaining non-judgmental awareness of one's thoughts, emotions, and sensations in the present moment. Microdosing has been reported to help individuals cultivate mindfulness by promoting a greater sense of self-awareness, emotional intelligence, and connection to the present moment. These effects may be related to the activation of serotonin receptors and modulation of the brain's default mode network (DMN), as previously discussed.

By fostering a greater sense of presence and self-awareness, microdosing may help individuals develop a more balanced relationship with their thoughts and emotions, reducing rumination and negative self-talk. This heightened mindfulness can lead to improved emotional regulation, stress reduction, and an overall sense of well-being.

Improving focus and concentration: In addition to enhancing mindfulness, microdosing has been associated with improved focus and concentration. Users often report increased mental clarity, the ability to maintain attention for longer periods, and heightened productivity. These cognitive benefits could be particularly valuable for individuals in intellectually demanding fields or those seeking to improve their performance in work, school, or other pursuits.

The mechanisms underlying these effects are not yet fully understood. However, they may be related to the interaction of psilocybin and psilocin with serotonin receptors, changes in brain connectivity, and increased neuroplasticity. By modulating brain activity and promoting a more flexible, open mental state, microdosing could help users overcome distractions, maintain focus, and engage more deeply with their tasks.

Integrating microdosing into a holistic mindfulness practice: For many individuals, microdosing serves as a complementary tool within a broader mindfulness practice, which may include meditation, yoga, journaling, or other self-reflection activities. By combining microdosing with these practices, users can create a holistic approach to self-improvement, mental health, and personal growth.

Case Studies and Anecdotes

While scientific research on microdosing is still in its early stages, numerous case studies and anecdotes provide valuable insights into the potential benefits and challenges associated with this practice. The following are a few examples of individual experiences with microdosing that highlight the diversity of outcomes and personal journeys.

Enhanced creativity and productivity: A graphic designer reported that microdosing psilocybin-containing mushrooms helped her overcome creative blocks and come up with innovative design concepts more effectively. She found that her ability to visualize complex ideas and generate novel solutions was significantly improved during her microdosing regimen, which ultimately led to increased productivity and satisfaction in her work.

Improved mood and emotional resilience: A software engineer suffering from chronic depression turned to microdosing as a potential alternative to traditional antidepressants. Over several weeks, he noticed a significant improvement in his mood, emotional resilience, and overall outlook on life. He reported feeling more connected to his emotions, experiencing greater self-awareness, and being better equipped to navigate challenging situations. This anecdotal account aligns with preliminary research suggesting that microdosing could hold promise as a treatment for depression and anxiety disorders.

Enhanced focus and attention: A graduate student struggling to maintain focus on her coursework decided to try microdosing to improve her attention and productivity. She found that during her microdosing regimen, she was better able to concentrate on complex tasks, retain information, and stay engaged with her studies for extended periods. This anecdote highlights the potential cognitive benefits of microdosing, including improved focus and concentration.

Unexpected challenges and negative experiences: While many anecdotal accounts describe positive outcomes, it is essential to acknowledge that microdosing may not be beneficial or suitable for everyone. One individual reported increased anxiety and paranoia during their microdosing regimen, ultimately deciding to discontinue the practice. This case emphasizes the importance of considering one's personal mental health history and risk factors before engaging in microdosing and being prepared to adjust or discontinue the practice if negative effects arise.

Managing chronic pain: A middle-aged woman with a history of chronic pain and fibromyalgia turned to microdosing in hopes of finding relief from her symptoms. Over several weeks, she reported a significant reduction in pain levels and an increased ability to engage in daily activities without being hindered by discomfort. This anecdote suggests that microdosing could potentially have a role in managing chronic pain, although more research is needed to understand the underlying mechanisms and confirm its efficacy.

Personal growth and self-awareness: A young professional engaged in microdosing as part of a broader self-improvement journey, which included practices like meditation, journaling, and yoga. He found that microdosing not only helped him cultivate greater self-awareness and emotional intelligence but also facilitated personal growth by encouraging introspection and a deeper understanding of his values, motivations, and goals. This account highlights the potential for microdosing to be integrated into a holistic approach to self-improvement and personal growth.

Improved athletic performance: An amateur athlete decided to try microdosing to enhance his focus and mental resilience during training and competitions. He reported that during his microdosing regimen, he experienced increased mental clarity, heightened concentration, and improved mind-body connection, which he believed contributed to enhanced athletic performance. This anecdote suggests that microdosing could potentially be of interest to athletes seeking a mental edge in their training and performance, although more research is needed to substantiate these claims.

Mixed experiences and the importance of personalization: A freelance writer began experimenting with microdosing to boost her creativity and productivity. While she initially noticed positive effects, such as increased focus and a greater ability to generate new ideas, she also experienced occasional bouts of increased anxiety and restlessness. This case highlights the importance of personalizing one's microdosing regimen, adjusting the dosage or frequency as needed, and being open to the possibility that the practice may not be universally beneficial or suitable for all individuals.

Alleviating symptoms of ADHD: An adult diagnosed with ADHD decided to try microdosing as an alternative to traditional stimulant medications. Over time, he reported increased focus, better impulse control, and an overall improvement in his ability to manage daily tasks and responsibilities. This anecdote suggests that microdosing might offer potential benefits for individuals with ADHD, although more research is needed to confirm its efficacy and understand the underlying mechanisms.

Supporting recovery from addiction: A woman recovering from alcohol addiction turned to microdosing as a complementary tool in her recovery process. She found that microdosing helped her manage cravings, reduce anxiety, and develop greater self-awareness and emotional resilience. While this personal account is encouraging, more research is needed to explore the potential role of microdosing in addiction treatment and recovery.

Overcoming writer's block: A novelist struggling with writer's block decided to try microdosing to stimulate her creativity and overcome her creative impasse. She reported that microdosing not only helped her generate new ideas and perspectives but also enabled her to approach her writing with renewed enthusiasm and motivation. This anecdote underscores the potential benefits of microdosing for individuals working in creative fields and facing similar challenges.

Coping with grief and loss: A man experiencing profound grief after the loss of a loved one turned to microdosing as a means of coping and finding emotional healing. He reported that microdosing helped him process his emotions more effectively, gain deeper insights into his feelings, and ultimately find a sense of acceptance and peace. While this account is inspiring, it's important to remember that individual experiences can vary, and microdosing may not be suitable or effective for everyone facing similar challenges.

Enhancing social skills and reducing social anxiety: A young man who experienced social anxiety and difficulty connecting with others decided to try microdosing to alleviate his symptoms. He reported increased self-confidence, improved communication skills, and greater ease in forming connections with others during his microdosing regimen. This anecdote suggests that microdosing might offer potential benefits for individuals struggling with social anxiety or seeking to enhance their social skills.

Boosting motivation and combating procrastination: A college student struggling with motivation and procrastination turned to microdosing as a potential solution. He found that microdosing helped him stay focused on his goals, prioritize tasks more effectively, and ultimately overcome his tendencies to procrastinate. This case highlights the potential benefits of microdosing for individuals seeking to improve their motivation and productivity.

Encouraging a deeper connection with nature: A nature enthusiast decided to incorporate microdosing into her outdoor adventures to deepen her connection with the natural world. She reported that microdosing heightened her senses, increased her appreciation for the beauty and intricacies of nature, and fostered a more profound sense of awe and wonder. This anecdote demonstrates the potential of microdosing to enhance one's connection with the environment and promote a greater appreciation for the natural world.

Navigating career transitions and personal growth: A professional facing a significant career transition began microdosing as a means of promoting self-reflection, clarity, and personal growth. He found that microdosing helped him gain new perspectives on his career path, identify his strengths and passions, and ultimately make more informed decisions about his future. This case emphasizes the potential of microdosing to facilitate personal growth and support individuals navigating significant life transitions.

These case studies and anecdotes provide a glimpse into the diverse experiences of individuals who have engaged in microdosing, highlighting the potential benefits and challenges associated with this practice. It is important to approach these accounts with curiosity and open-mindedness while recognizing that individual experiences can vary widely. As the scientific understanding of microdosing continues to evolve, personal accounts will remain an essential source of information and inspiration for those considering this practice.

Microdosing for Improved Athletic Performance

The world of athletic performance is constantly evolving, with athletes and fitness enthusiasts seeking innovative methods to optimize their physical capabilities, boost recovery, and gain a competitive edge. In recent years, microdosing psychedelic mushrooms has emerged as a cutting-edge approach to enhancing athletic performance in ways that extend beyond traditional training and nutrition techniques.

In this chapter, we delve into the potential benefits of microdosing for athletes and fitness enthusiasts, exploring how this practice can amplify physical and mental stamina, improve mind-body connection and coordination, and accelerate recovery by reducing stress. By examining the science and anecdotal evidence behind these performance-enhancing effects, we aim to provide a comprehensive understanding of how microdosing can transform the way we approach sports and physical activity.

Whether you are a professional athlete seeking new ways to elevate your performance, a fitness enthusiast looking to overcome plateaus, or simply someone interested in the potential benefits of microdosing in the realm of athletic performance, this chapter offers valuable insights and guidance on harnessing the power of psychedelic mushrooms to reach new heights in your physical pursuits.

Enhancing Physical and Mental Stamina

Microdosing with psychedelic mushrooms may provide athletes with a competitive edge by enhancing their physical and mental stamina. This section discusses how microdosing can contribute to increased energy levels, focus, and mental endurance, allowing athletes to optimize their training and push through barriers during demanding physical activities.

Increased energy levels: Some anecdotal reports suggest that microdosing may result in increased energy levels, giving athletes the extra boost they need to tackle their workouts and maintain high-intensity performance. This energy boost may stem from the stimulating effects of the active compounds in psychedelic mushrooms, such as psilocybin and psilocin, which can improve alertness and overall vitality.

Improved focus and concentration: Microdosing has been associated with enhanced focus and concentration, which are essential to athletic performance. The ability to maintain attention on a specific task, such as running a race or executing a complex movement, can be the difference between success and failure in competitive sports. By promoting mental clarity and reducing distractions, microdosing may help athletes stay focused during training sessions and competitions.

Mental endurance and resilience: In addition to physical stamina, mental endurance plays a crucial role in athletic performance. Athletes often face mental barriers that can limit their potentials, such as performance anxiety, self-doubt, or the challenge of staying motivated during long and grueling training sessions. Microdosing may help athletes develop mental resilience by boosting mood, reducing anxiety, and fostering a positive mindset. This can translate into increased motivation, determination, and the ability to push through mental barriers that might otherwise impede performance.

Flow state and peak performance: Microdosing has been linked to the experience of "flow," a state of complete immersion in an activity characterized by heightened focus, creativity, and a sense of effortless performance. Athletes often describe flow states as being "in the zone," where their movements feel natural and seamless, and their performance reaches its peak. By facilitating access to flow states, microdosing may help athletes unlock their full potential and achieve optimal performance levels during training and competition.

In conclusion, microdosing with psychedelic mushrooms may offer athletes a unique opportunity to enhance their physical and mental stamina. By increasing energy levels, improving focus and concentration, fostering mental resilience, and promoting access to flow states, microdosing may help athletes optimize their training and achieve peak performance in their chosen disciplines.

Boosting Mind-body Connection And Coordination

Microdosing with psychedelic mushrooms may provide athletes with benefits beyond mental and physical stamina, such as enhancing the mind-body connection and improving coordination. This section explores how microdosing can contribute to better body awareness, fine-tuning of motor skills, and overall improved athletic performance across various disciplines.

Enhanced body awareness: Microdosing has been associated with an increased sense of self-awareness, which can extend to a heightened awareness of one's body. This improved body awareness can help athletes become more in tune with their physical sensations, muscle movements, and the subtle nuances of their technique. As a result, athletes may be better equipped to make adjustments to their form, leading to more efficient and effective movement patterns.

Improved coordination and motor skills: Athletic performance often relies on precise coordination and well-honed motor skills. Anecdotal reports and some preliminary research suggest that microdosing may have a positive impact on these aspects of athletic performance. Enhancing the mind-body connection, microdosing may help athletes refine their motor skills and improve their coordination, ultimately leading to better execution of complex movements and techniques.

Adaptability and learning new skills: The potential cognitive benefits of microdosing, such as increased focus and creativity, may also extend to learning new skills and adapting to new challenges in the athletic context. Athletes who are better able to adapt and learn new techniques may have a competitive advantage, as they can continually refine their performance and stay ahead of their competitors.

Enhanced proprioception and balance: Proprioception, or the sense of one's body position in space, is a crucial aspect of athletic performance, particularly in activities that require balance and agility. Some anecdotal evidence suggests that microdosing may enhance proprioception, allowing athletes to improve their balance and spatial awareness. This could be particularly beneficial for athletes involved in sports such as gymnastics, dance, or martial arts.

Microdosing with psychedelic mushrooms may offer athletes a unique opportunity to boost their mind-body connection and coordination. By enhancing body awareness, improving coordination and motor skills, promoting adaptability, and potentially increasing proprioception and balance, microdosing may help athletes refine their performance and excel in their chosen disciplines. However, more research is needed to fully understand the extent of these potential benefits and to establish guidelines for safe and responsible use in athletic contexts.

Accelerating Recovery and Reducing Stress

Recovery is a crucial aspect of athletic performance, as it allows the body to heal and adapt after strenuous workouts or competitions. Microdosing with psychedelic mushrooms may play a role in promoting faster recovery and reducing stress, helping athletes maintain peak performance levels and prevent injuries.

Alleviating stress and promoting relaxation: Athletes often face high levels of stress, both physical and mental, which can impede recovery and increase the risk of injury. Some anecdotal reports suggest that microdosing may help reduce stress and promote relaxation by regulating mood and fostering a sense of calm and well-being. By managing stress more effectively, athletes may be better equipped to recover from intense training sessions and maintain their overall mental and physical health.

Reducing inflammation and promoting healing: Inflammation is a natural response to physical stress and plays a role in the recovery process; however, excessive inflammation can slow down healing and contribute to chronic pain or injury. Preliminary research on psychedelics, including psilocybin, suggests that they may have anti-inflammatory properties. This could potentially help athletes manage inflammation, promote faster healing, and reduce the risk of overuse injuries or chronic pain.

Improving sleep quality: Sleep is a critical component of recovery, as it allows the body to repair and regenerate. Microdosing has been associated with improved sleep quality in some anecdotal accounts, which may help athletes optimize their recovery process. By promoting restful and restorative sleep, microdosing may contribute to better overall recovery and improved athletic performance.

Boosting mood and emotional resilience: Athletes often face emotional challenges, such as performance anxiety, self-doubt, or the pressure to succeed. Microdosing may help athletes develop emotional resilience by enhancing mood, reducing anxiety, and promoting a more positive mindset. This and can lead to a more balanced emotional state, which may be beneficial for recovery and maintaining motivation during demanding training periods.

Supporting mindfulness and self-care: Microdosing has been linked to increased mindfulness and self-awareness, which can help athletes develop a greater sense of self-care and prioritize their recovery needs. By becoming more attuned to their bodies and emotional states, athletes can make more informed decisions about when to rest, seek support, or modify their training programs to optimize recovery and prevent burnout.

In conclusion, microdosing with psychedelic mushrooms may offer athletes a unique opportunity to accelerate their recovery process and reduce stress. By alleviating stress, reducing inflammation, improving sleep quality, boosting mood and emotional resilience, and promoting mindfulness and self-care, microdosing may help athletes maintain peak performance levels and minimize the risk of injury.

Microdosing for Emotional Well-being

In a world where emotional well-being is increasingly recognized as a vital component of overall health, people are continuously seeking effective strategies to manage stress, anxiety, and depression. Microdosing psychedelic mushrooms has emerged as a powerful tool that holds the potential to transform emotional well-being, promoting balance and resilience in the face of life's challenges.

This chapter delves into the realm of microdosing for emotional well-being, exploring its potential benefits in addressing anxiety, depression, and stress. We will discuss how microdosing can boost mood and emotional resilience, as well as its potential to enhance mindfulness practices, leading to a more centered and peaceful state of mind. By examining scientific research and personal accounts, we aim to provide a comprehensive understanding of the impact microdosing can have on emotional health.

Whether you are struggling with emotional challenges, seeking to cultivate greater self-awareness, or simply curious about the potential benefits of microdosing for emotional well-being, this chapter offers valuable insights and guidance on how to harness the power of psychedelic mushrooms to foster a more balanced and fulfilling emotional life.

Addressing Anxiety, Depression, and Stress

Microdosing has attracted significant interest as a potential alternative or complementary approach to addressing anxiety, depression, and stress. While research is still in its early stages, anecdotal evidence and preliminary findings suggest that microdosing may offer some benefits for individuals experiencing these mental health challenges. This section explores the potential mechanisms, benefits, and considerations associated with microdosing for anxiety, depression, and stress.

Potential mechanisms: Microdosing's effects on anxiety, depression, and stress could be related to its interaction with serotonin receptors in the brain. Psilocybin and psilocin, the active compounds in psychedelic mushrooms, have been shown to bind to serotonin receptors, particularly the 5-HT2A receptor. This interaction may lead to increased neuroplasticity, enhanced mood, and improved emotional regulation. Additionally, microdosing has been associated with modulation of the default mode network (DMN), which is involved in self-referential thinking, rumination, and introspection. Disruption of the DMN may help individuals break free from negative thought patterns and promote a more balanced mental state.

Potential benefits: Many individuals who have tried microdosing for anxiety, depression, and stress report improvements in mood, emotional resilience, and overall well-being. Some anecdotal accounts describe reduced symptoms of anxiety, a greater ability to cope with stress, and a more positive outlook on life. Others mention enhanced self-awareness, increased emotional intelligence, and a deeper connection to the present moment, which can contribute to improved mental health.

While anecdotal evidence is encouraging, it is essential to recognize that scientific research on microdosing for anxiety, depression, and stress is still in its infancy. More rigorous, controlled studies are needed to determine the efficacy, safety, and optimal protocols for microdosing in this context.

Microdosing should be approached with caution and responsibility, and individuals should be prepared to adjust or discontinue their regimen if negative effects arise. Microdosing holds promise as a potential tool for addressing anxiety, depression, and stress, but more research is needed to fully understand its efficacy and safety. Anecdotal evidence provides valuable insights into the potential benefits and challenges associated with microdosing for mental health, but it is crucial for individuals to consider their personal circumstances, goals, and risk factors when exploring this practice.

Boosting Mood and Emotional Resilience

Microdosing has gained attention as a potential tool for boosting mood and enhancing emotional resilience. By promoting a more balanced mental state, microdosing may help individuals cultivate a greater sense of well-being and navigate life's challenges more effectively. This section will discuss the potential mechanisms, benefits, and considerations associated with microdosing for mood enhancement and emotional resilience.

Potential mechanisms: The mood-enhancing effects of microdosing may be related to its interaction with serotonin receptors in the brain. Psilocybin and psilocin, the active compounds in psychedelic mushrooms, bind to serotonin receptors, particularly the 5-HT2A receptor. This interaction can lead to increased neuroplasticity, which supports the brain's ability to adapt and change in response to new experiences and challenges. Additionally, microdosing has been associated with modulation of the default mode network (DMN), which plays a role in self-referential thinking, rumination, and introspection. By disrupting the DMN, microdosing may help individuals break free from negative thought patterns and cultivate a more balanced and positive mindset.

Potential benefits: Anecdotal evidence and preliminary research suggest that microdosing can lead to improvements in mood, emotional resilience, and overall well-being. Individuals who have tried microdosing often report increased self-awareness, enhanced emotional intelligence, and a greater connection to the present moment. These factors can contribute to improved mental health, a more positive outlook on life, and a better ability to cope with stress and adversity.

Some anecdotal accounts describe reduced symptoms of depression and anxiety, as well as a heightened sense of joy, gratitude, and wonder. Others mention increased motivation, energy, and optimism, which can lead to greater satisfaction and fulfillment in various aspects of life.

Mindfulness Practices and Microdosing

The combination of mindfulness practices and microdosing has attracted interest as a means of enhancing personal growth, self-awareness, and mental well-being. Both approaches can support individuals in developing greater focus, emotional regulation, and resilience. This section explores the potential synergies, benefits, and considerations associated with integrating mindfulness practices and microdosing.

Potential synergies: Mindfulness practices, such as meditation, yoga, and breathwork, emphasize being fully present and engaged in the current moment, cultivating awareness and acceptance of thoughts and emotions without judgment. Microdosing can potentially enhance these practices by promoting a heightened sense of self-awareness, increased sensitivity to internal experiences, and a deeper connection to the present moment.

The combination of mindfulness practices and microdosing may help individuals break free from negative thought patterns, improve emotional regulation, and develop a greater sense of overall well-being. Furthermore, both approaches can support neuroplasticity, which is the brain's ability to adapt and change in response to new experiences and challenges.

Potential benefits: Integrating mindfulness practices and microdosing may offer several benefits, including:

- Improved focus and concentration during mindfulness practices, allowing for deeper and more meaningful experiences.
- Enhanced emotional intelligence and self-awareness, supporting better understanding and management of emotions.
- Greater resilience and adaptability, empowering individuals to navigate life's challenges more effectively.
- Reduced symptoms of anxiety and depression, fostering a more positive and balanced mental state.
- Increased creativity and problem-solving skills, which can contribute to personal growth and fulfillment.

It is important to note that research on the combined effects of mindfulness practices and microdosing is limited, and more studies are needed to confirm these potential benefits.

The combination of mindfulness practices and microdosing holds promise as a potential tool for personal growth and mental well-being, but more research is needed to fully understand its efficacy and safety. Anecdotal evidence provides valuable insights into the potential benefits and challenges associated with this integrated approach, but it is crucial for individuals to consider their personal circumstances, goals, and risk factors when exploring these practices.

Microdosing for Personal Growth and Spiritual Exploration

In our ever-changing world, the pursuit of personal growth and spiritual exploration has become increasingly important for many individuals seeking deeper meaning, self-awareness, and a more profound connection with themselves and the world around them. Microdosing psychedelic mushrooms has emerged as a promising tool for enhancing personal growth and facilitating spiritual exploration in a nuanced and accessible manner.

In this chapter, we delve into the captivating realm of microdosing for personal growth and spiritual exploration. We will discuss how microdosing can help expand self-awareness and introspection, nurture a deeper connection to the self and the world, and even integrate seamlessly into various spiritual practices. Drawing from both scientific research and personal experiences, we will shed light on the transformative potential of microdosing in facilitating self-discovery and spiritual growth.

Whether you are on a spiritual journey, seeking to cultivate a greater understanding of your inner self, or simply curious about the potential benefits of microdosing for personal growth and spiritual exploration, this chapter offers valuable insights and guidance on how to harness the power of psychedelic mushrooms to embark on a transformative path of self-discovery and spiritual awakening.

Expanding Self-awareness and Introspection

Microdosing has gained attention as a potential tool for expanding self-awareness and promoting introspection, supporting personal growth and a deeper understanding of one's thoughts, emotions, and behaviors. By fostering a more nuanced and compassionate perspective on the self, microdosing may help individuals navigate life's challenges and cultivate greater mental well-being. This section explores the potential mechanisms, benefits, and considerations associated with microdosing for self-awareness and introspection.

Potential mechanisms: The effects of microdosing on self-awareness and introspection may be linked to its interaction with serotonin receptors in the brain. Psilocybin and psilocin, the active compounds in psychedelic mushrooms, bind to serotonin receptors, particularly the 5-HT2A receptor. This interaction can lead to increased neuroplasticity, supporting the brain's ability to adapt and change in response to new experiences and challenges.

Additionally, microdosing has been associated with modulation of the default mode network (DMN), which plays a role in self-referential thinking, rumination, and introspection. By disrupting the DMN, microdosing may help individuals break free from negative thought patterns, gain new perspectives on their thoughts and emotions, and ultimately cultivate a more balanced and compassionate understanding of the self.

Potential benefits: Anecdotal evidence and preliminary research suggest that microdosing can contribute to increased self-awareness, introspection, and overall well-being. Individuals who have tried microdosing often report:

- Enhanced emotional intelligence, allowing for a better understanding and management of emotions.
- Greater insight into personal values, motivations, and strengths, which can inform personal growth and decision-making.
- Improved empathy and compassion towards oneself and others, fostering healthier relationships and social connections.

- A deeper connection to the present moment, promoting mindfulness and a more balanced mental state.
- Reduced symptoms of anxiety and depression, supporting a more positive outlook on life.

In conclusion, microdosing holds promise as a potential tool for expanding self-awareness and promoting introspection, but more research is needed to fully understand its efficacy and safety. Anecdotal evidence provides valuable insights into the potential benefits and challenges associated with microdosing for personal growth and mental well-being, but it is crucial for individuals to consider their personal circumstances, goals, and risk factors when exploring this practice.

Nurturing a Deeper Connection to the Self and the World

Microdosing has gained interest as a potential tool for nurturing a deeper connection to the self and the world around us. By fostering a heightened sense of awareness, compassion, and empathy, microdosing may help individuals cultivate a greater sense of well-being, interconnectedness, and harmony with their environment. This section explores the potential mechanisms, benefits, and considerations associated with microdosing for deepening connections to the self and the world.

Potential mechanisms: The effects of microdosing on deepening connections may be related to its interaction with serotonin receptors in the brain. Psilocybin and psilocin, the active compounds in psychedelic mushrooms, bind to serotonin receptors, particularly the 5-HT2A receptor. This interaction can lead to increased neuroplasticity, which supports the brain's ability to adapt and change in response to new experiences and challenges.

Additionally, microdosing has been associated with modulation of the default mode network (DMN), which is involved in self-referential thinking, rumination, and introspection. By disrupting the DMN, microdosing may help individuals break free from negative thought patterns and cultivate a more balanced, compassionate, and connected perspective on themselves and their environment.

Potential benefits: Anecdotal evidence and preliminary research suggest that microdosing can contribute to deepening connections to the self and the world, with potential benefits including:

- Increased self-awareness, introspection, and emotional intelligence, which can support personal growth and self-compassion.
- Enhanced empathy and compassion towards others, fostering healthier relationships and social connections.
- A heightened sense of interconnectedness and appreciation for the natural world, promoting environmental awareness and stewardship.
- Improved mindfulness and presence, allowing for a deeper connection to the present moment and a more balanced mental state.
- Reduced feelings of isolation, loneliness, and alienation, supporting overall mental well-being and a sense of belonging.

In conclusion, microdosing holds promise as a potential tool for deepening connections to the self and the world, but more research is needed to fully understand its efficacy and safety. Anecdotal evidence provides valuable insights into the potential benefits and challenges associated with microdosing for personal growth and interconnectedness, but it is crucial for individuals to consider their personal circumstances, goals, and risk factors when exploring this practice.

Integrating Microdosing into Spiritual Practices

Microdosing has attracted interest as a potential tool for enhancing spiritual practices, promoting personal growth, self-discovery, and a deeper connection to the transcendent. By fostering a heightened sense of awareness and presence, microdosing may help individuals cultivate a greater sense of well-being and spiritual connection. This section explores the potential mechanisms, benefits, and considerations associated with integrating microdosing into spiritual practices.

Potential mechanisms: The effects of microdosing on spiritual practices may be related to its interaction with serotonin receptors in the brain. Psilocybin and psilocin, the active compounds in psychedelic mushrooms, bind to serotonin receptors, particularly the 5-HT2A receptor. This interaction can lead to increased neuroplasticity, which supports the brain's ability to adapt and change in response to new experiences and challenges.

Additionally, microdosing has been associated with modulation of the default mode network (DMN), which plays a role in self-referential thinking, rumination, and introspection. By disrupting the DMN, microdosing may help individuals break free from negative thought patterns, gain new perspectives, and cultivate a more balanced and connected understanding of themselves and the world.

Potential benefits: Integrating microdosing into spiritual practices may offer several benefits, including:

- Enhanced presence and focus during meditation, prayer, or other contemplative practices, allowing for deeper and more meaningful experiences.

- Heightened self-awareness, introspection, and emotional intelligence, which can support personal growth, self-compassion, and spiritual development.
- A sense of interconnectedness and unity with others, the natural world, and the transcendent, fostering a greater appreciation for the sacred and the divine.
- Improved creativity and openness, which can contribute to a richer and more diverse spiritual journey.
- Reduced feelings of isolation, loneliness, and alienation, supporting overall mental well-being and a sense of belonging to a larger spiritual community.

In conclusion, the integration of microdosing into spiritual practices holds promise as a potential tool for personal growth and spiritual development, but more research is needed to fully understand its efficacy and safety. Anecdotal evidence provides valuable insights into the potential benefits and challenges associated with this integrated approach, but it is crucial for individuals to consider their personal circumstances, goals, and risk factors when exploring these practices.

Microdosing for Better Sleep

In today's fast-paced world, quality sleep has become a precious commodity, with many people struggling to achieve restorative rest and a balanced sleep pattern. As the importance of sleep for our overall health and well-being becomes increasingly recognized, novel approaches to enhancing sleep quality are being explored. One such approach that has gained attention in recent years is microdosing psychedelic mushrooms, which has shown potential in promoting better sleep and fostering a healthier relationship with our nightly rest.

In this chapter, we delve into the world of microdosing for better sleep, examining how this practice can help regulate sleep patterns, balance mood, and stress levels, and even enhance dream recall and lucidity. By exploring scientific research and anecdotal evidence, we aim to provide a comprehensive understanding of the impact microdosing can have on our sleep and how it can contribute to a more restful and rejuvenating slumber.

Whether you are struggling with sleep issues, seeking to deepen your understanding of your dreams, or simply curious about the potential benefits of microdosing for sleep, this chapter offers valuable insights and guidance on how to harness the power of psychedelic mushrooms to transform your nightly rest and improve your overall sleep quality.

Regulating Sleep Patterns

Sleep is a vital aspect of maintaining optimal health and well-being. Microdosing with psychedelic mushrooms has the potential to regulate sleep patterns, address sleep issues such as insomnia, and improve overall sleep quality. This section discusses how microdosing may contribute to enhanced restorative sleep, leading to improved physical and mental health.

Addressing sleep issues: Many individuals struggle with sleep issues, including insomnia, which can negatively impact their daily functioning and overall quality of life. Anecdotal reports suggest that microdosing may help regulate sleep patterns by promoting relaxation and reducing stress, which are often factors contributing to sleep problems. By addressing these underlying issues, microdosing may help individuals fall asleep more easily and experience more restful sleep.

Promoting a consistent sleep schedule: A consistent sleep schedule is essential for maintaining a healthy sleep cycle and ensuring the body receives adequate rest. Microdosing may help individuals establish a more consistent sleep schedule by promoting a sense of calm and relaxation, making it easier for them to fall asleep at a regular time each night. This consistency can contribute to a more balanced circadian rhythm and improved overall sleep quality.

Enhancing sleep quality: Sleep quality is just as important as sleep quantity, as it allows the body and mind to fully recover and recharge during the night. Anecdotal evidence suggests that microdosing may improve sleep quality by increasing the time spent in deep sleep and REM sleep, which are crucial for physical and mental restoration. Enhanced sleep quality may result in individuals waking up feeling more refreshed, alert, and energized, positively impacting their daily functioning and well-being.

Reducing sleep disruptions: Sleep disruptions, such as frequent awakenings during the night or difficulty falling back asleep, can prevent individuals from receiving adequate rest. Microdosing may help reduce sleep disruptions by promoting relaxation, reducing anxiety, and addressing other factors that may contribute to interrupted sleep. By reducing these disruptions, individuals may experience more continuous and restorative sleep.

Microdosing with psychedelic mushrooms may offer individuals a unique opportunity to regulate their sleep patterns and improve overall sleep quality. By addressing sleep issues, promoting a consistent sleep schedule, enhancing sleep quality, and reducing sleep disruptions, microdosing may contribute to better physical and mental health.

Balancing Mood and Stress Reduction

Mood and stress levels can have a significant impact on sleep quality, making it essential to address these factors in order to improve sleep patterns. Microdosing with psychedelic mushrooms may offer benefits in balancing mood and reducing stress, creating a more conducive environment for healthy sleep. This section explores the potential effects of microdosing on mood regulation and stress reduction, and how these factors may contribute to improved sleep quality.

Alleviating anxiety and depression: Anecdotal reports and preliminary research suggest that microdosing may have a positive impact on mood, potentially helping to alleviate symptoms of anxiety and depression. By reducing these symptoms, microdosing may promote relaxation and a sense of well-being, making it easier for individuals to fall asleep and stay asleep throughout the night.

Reducing stress levels: Stress is a common factor that can negatively affect sleep quality, as it may make it difficult for individuals to relax and wind down before bed. Microdosing may help reduce stress levels by promoting a sense of calm and inducing a more positive emotional state. This stress reduction may help individuals feel more relaxed and better prepared for sleep, leading to improved sleep quality and overall well-being.

Enhancing emotional resilience: Microdosing has been associated with increased emotional resilience, which may help individuals cope more effectively with daily stressors and maintain a more balanced emotional state. This enhanced resilience can contribute to better sleep quality, as individuals may be less likely to experience sleep disruptions caused by stress or negative emotions.

Promoting relaxation and mindfulness: Microdosing has been linked to increased mindfulness and relaxation, both of which can play a role in promoting healthy sleep. By fostering a sense of calm and presence, microdosing may help individuals develop a more relaxed state of mind, making it easier to let go of stress and tension before bed. This increased relaxation can facilitate the transition into sleep and improve overall sleep quality.

Microdosing with psychedelic mushrooms may offer individuals a unique opportunity to balance their mood and reduce stress, which can contribute to improved sleep quality. By alleviating anxiety and depression, reducing stress levels, enhancing emotional resilience, and promoting relaxation and mindfulness, microdosing may help create a more conducive environment for restorative sleep. However, more research is needed to fully understand the extent of these potential benefits and to establish guidelines for safe and responsible use in the context of sleep improvement.

Enhancing Dream Recall and Lucidity

Dreams play a crucial role in our mental well-being, providing a space for processing emotions, memories, and experiences. Microdosing with psychedelic mushrooms has been associated with enhanced dream recall and lucid dreaming, which could contribute to improved sleep quality and personal growth through the exploration of one's inner world during sleep. This section discusses the potential effects of microdosing on dream recall and lucidity, and how these factors may impact sleep quality and overall well-being.

Improving dream recall: Anecdotal reports suggest that microdosing may enhance dream recall, making it easier for individuals to remember their dreams upon waking. This improved dream recall can provide valuable insights into one's subconscious mind, offering opportunities for self-reflection, problem-solving, and personal growth. By facilitating a deeper connection to the dream world, microdosing may promote a greater understanding of one's inner thoughts and emotions, ultimately contributing to better mental health and well-being.

Promoting lucid dreaming: Lucid dreaming is the phenomenon in which an individual becomes aware that they are dreaming and may gain some control over the dream's content. Some anecdotal accounts and preliminary research indicate that microdosing may promote lucid dreaming by enhancing self-awareness and mindfulness, making it more likely for individuals to recognize when they are dreaming. Lucid dreaming can offer unique opportunities for personal exploration, creativity, and problem-solving, potentially leading to greater self-discovery and personal growth.

Enhancing sleep quality and well-being: The potential effects of microdosing on dream recall and lucidity may contribute to improved sleep quality and overall well-being. By fostering a more meaningful connection to the dream world, microdosing may help individuals process emotions, memories, and experiences more effectively, promoting mental and emotional balance. This improved sleep quality and enhanced dream experience can lead to a greater sense of well-being and overall life satisfaction.

Exploring therapeutic potential: Enhanced dream recall and lucid dreaming have been associated with potential therapeutic benefits, including the processing of traumatic experiences, the resolution of emotional conflicts, and the development of coping strategies. The potential effects of microdosing on dream recall and lucidity may open new avenues for exploring the therapeutic potential of dreams in the context of personal growth and mental health treatment.

Microdosing with psychedelic mushrooms may offer individuals a unique opportunity to enhance dream recall and promote lucid dreaming, potentially leading to improved sleep quality, personal growth, and overall well-being. By improving dream recall, promoting lucid dreaming, and exploring the therapeutic potential of dreams, microdosing may contribute to a greater understanding of one's inner world and emotional landscape.

Microdosing Safely and Responsibly

As the practice of microdosing psychedelic mushrooms continues to gain traction and acceptance, it is essential to recognize the importance of engaging in this powerful tool safely and responsibly. While microdosing has been shown to provide numerous benefits, it is not without potential risks and considerations. Being informed and mindful of these aspects is critical to ensure a positive and meaningful microdosing experience.

In this chapter, we will discuss the various aspects of microdosing safely and responsibly, covering topics such as legal considerations, potential risks, contraindications, precautions, and the importance of building a support network and self-monitoring. Our aim is to provide a comprehensive understanding of the safety and responsibility concerns surrounding microdosing, empowering you to make informed decisions and minimize potential risks while maximizing the benefits of this transformative practice.

This chapter will serve as a valuable resource for ensuring that your microdosing journey is undertaken with safety, responsibility, and a deep respect for the transformative potential of these powerful natural allies.

Legal Considerations and Potential Risks

Understanding the legal considerations and potential risks associated with microdosing psychedelic mushrooms is essential for those considering this practice. While the potential benefits of microdosing are increasingly recognized, it is crucial to weigh them against the legal implications and possible risks.

Legal status of psychedelic mushrooms: The legal status of psychedelic mushrooms varies by country and region:

- In the United States, psilocybin and psilocin are classified as Schedule I substances under the Controlled Substances Act, making the possession, cultivation, and sale of psychedelic mushrooms illegal at the federal level. However, some cities and states have decriminalized the possession of psilocybin mushrooms for personal use.
- In Canada, psilocybin and psilocin are listed as Schedule III substances under the Controlled Drugs and Substances Act. However, exceptions have been made for certain medical and religious purposes.
- In some European countries, such as the Netherlands, the sale of "magic truffles" containing psilocybin is legal, while mushroom sales remain prohibited.

It is essential to be aware of and comply with local laws and regulations regarding psychedelic mushrooms in your jurisdiction.

Potential risks: There are several potential risks associated with microdosing psychedelic mushrooms, including:

- Physical risks: While psychedelic mushrooms are considered relatively safe, some individuals may experience adverse physical reactions, such as nausea, dizziness, or increased heart rate.
- Psychological risks: Microdosing may exacerbate pre-existing mental health conditions or induce anxiety, paranoia, or mood disturbances in susceptible individuals.
- Legal risks: The possession, cultivation, or sale of psychedelic mushrooms may result in legal consequences, such as fines, arrest, or imprisonment, depending on local laws and regulations.

- Employment risks: Microdosing could lead to a positive drug test or conflicts with workplace policies, potentially resulting in job loss or other professional consequences.

Mitigating risks: To minimize potential risks associated with microdosing, consider the following steps:

- Know the law: Familiarize yourself with local laws and regulations regarding psychedelic mushrooms and act accordingly to minimize legal risks.
- Consult a healthcare professional: If you have a pre-existing medical condition or are taking medications, consult with a healthcare professional before beginning a microdosing regimen.
- Start with a low dose: Begin with a low dose and gradually increase as needed to minimize potential side effects and find the optimal dosage for your needs.
- Follow a microdosing schedule: Adhering to a microdosing schedule can help prevent the development of tolerance and minimize potential side effects.
- Practice harm reduction: Use accurate dosing and measurement techniques, source mushrooms responsibly, and prioritize self-care to minimize potential risks.

Understanding the legal considerations and potential risks associated with microdosing psychedelic mushrooms is essential for those considering this practice. By being aware of local laws and regulations, weighing the potential benefits against the risks, and taking steps to mitigate these risks, individuals can make informed decisions about whether microdosing is the right choice for them.

Contraindications and Precautions

Before engaging in microdosing with psychedelic mushrooms, it is crucial to consider contraindications and precautions to ensure safety and minimize potential adverse effects. Certain medical conditions, medications, and personal factors may make microdosing inappropriate or potentially harmful.

Medical contraindications: Some medical conditions may make microdosing inadvisable or potentially dangerous:

- Mental health disorders: Individuals with a history of psychosis, schizophrenia, bipolar disorder, or severe anxiety should approach microdosing with caution, as it may exacerbate symptoms or trigger episodes.
- Cardiovascular issues: Psychedelic mushrooms can cause an increase in heart rate and blood pressure. Those with a history of heart disease or hypertension should consult with a healthcare professional before microdosing.
- Pregnancy and breastfeeding: The safety of microdosing during pregnancy and breastfeeding is not well established. It is generally recommended to avoid microdosing during these periods to protect the health of the mother and child.

Medication interactions: Some medications may interact negatively with the active compounds in psychedelic mushrooms:

- Selective serotonin reuptake inhibitors (SSRIs) and other antidepressants: Combining SSRIs with psychedelic mushrooms may reduce the effectiveness of microdosing due to the shared action on serotonin receptors. There is also a small risk of developing serotonin syndrome, a potentially life-threatening condition.

- Monoamine oxidase inhibitors (MAOIs): Combining MAOIs with psychedelic mushrooms may increase the risk of serotonin syndrome or potentiate the effects of psilocybin, leading to an unexpectedly strong reaction.
- Blood pressure medications: Combining blood pressure medications with psychedelic mushrooms may lead to unpredictable effects on blood pressure and heart rate.

Always consult with a healthcare professional before starting a microdosing regimen if you are taking any medications.

Personal precautions: Individual factors and personal circumstances may impact the safety and effectiveness of microdosing:
- Age: Adolescents and young adults should approach microdosing with caution due to ongoing brain development and the potential for long-term effects on mental health.
- Substance use history: Those with a history of substance abuse or addiction should be cautious when microdosing, as it may trigger cravings or impede recovery.
- Set and setting: Ensure that you are in a comfortable and supportive environment when microdosing to minimize potential anxiety and maximize the benefits of the experience.

General advice for safe microdosing: To ensure a safe and beneficial microdosing experience, consider the following tips:

- Start with a low dose: Begin with a low dose and gradually increase as needed to find your optimal dosage while minimizing potential side effects.
- Follow a microdosing schedule: Adhering to a microdosing schedule can help prevent the development of tolerance and minimize potential side effects.

- Keep a journal: Record your experiences, dosage, and any side effects to help refine your microdosing regimen and maximize the benefits.
- Listen to your body: Pay attention to how your body and mind react to microdosing, and adjust your dosage or schedule accordingly to ensure a safe and positive experience.

Considering contraindications and precautions is essential for a safe and effective microdosing experience with psychedelic mushrooms. By being aware of potential medical contraindications, medication interactions, and personal factors, and following general advice for safe microdosing, individuals can minimize potential risks and maximize the potential benefits of their microdosing journey.

Building a Support Network and Self-monitoring

Having a support network and engaging in self-monitoring are essential aspects of a successful and safe microdosing journey. A support network can provide guidance, encouragement, and a safe space to share experiences and insights. Self-monitoring helps track the effects of microdosing and facilitates adjustments to dosage or schedule as needed.

Importance of a support network: A support network can play a crucial role in the microdosing journey for several reasons:

- Guidance and advice: Those with experience in microdosing can provide valuable insights, recommendations, and tips to help navigate the process.
- Emotional support: Sharing experiences, challenges, and triumphs with like-minded individuals can provide encouragement and motivation.

- Safety net: A support network can offer assistance in case of unexpected side effects or difficulties during the microdosing process.

Finding support: There are several ways to build a support network for microdosing:

- Personal connections: Reach out to friends or family members who are knowledgeable about or experienced with microdosing. They can provide personal insights and a familiar source of support.
- Online forums and communities: Join online forums or social media groups dedicated to microdosing, where individuals can share experiences, ask questions, and offer advice. Examples include Reddit's r/microdosing community or specialized Facebook groups.
- Local meetups and events: Attend local meetups, workshops, or conferences related to psychedelics and microdosing to connect with others who share similar interests and experiences.
- Professional support: Consult with healthcare professionals, therapists, or specialized coaches experienced in working with psychedelics to receive guidance and support tailored to your unique needs.

Self-monitoring strategies: Engaging in self-monitoring helps track the effects of microdosing and enables adjustments to dosage or schedule as needed. Some effective self-monitoring strategies include:

- Journaling: Keep a detailed journal of your microdosing experiences, noting the dosage, timing, effects, side effects, and any insights gained. This can help identify patterns and facilitate adjustments to your microdosing regimen.

- Mood tracking: Use mood tracking apps or create a simple chart to monitor changes in mood, energy, and well-being throughout the microdosing process.
- Cognitive assessments: Perform regular cognitive assessments using online tools or apps to evaluate potential changes in cognitive function, memory, or problem-solving abilities.
- Goal setting and reflection: Set specific, measurable goals for your microdosing journey and regularly reflect on your progress towards these goals. Adjust your dosage or schedule to optimize the benefits and minimize side effects.

Building a support network and self-monitoring are vital to a successful and safe microdosing journey. By connecting with others, seeking guidance, and tracking the effects of microdosing, individuals can optimize their experience and maximize the potential benefits of this practice.

Integration and Reflection

Embarking on a microdosing journey with psychedelic mushrooms is more than just an exploration of the immediate benefits it may bring to various aspects of our lives. To truly harness the power of microdosing, it is crucial to integrate the insights, shifts in perspective, and personal growth experienced during this process into our everyday lives. Reflection and integration are key components in making lasting and meaningful changes, turning the lessons learned through microdosing into tangible improvements in our well-being, relationships, and overall life satisfaction.

In this chapter, we will explore the importance of integration and reflection in the context of microdosing psychedelic mushrooms. We will discuss strategies for tracking and evaluating your microdosing experiences, methods for integrating the insights gained into your daily life, and guidance on when to take breaks or stop microdosing altogether. By providing a roadmap for reflection and integration, this chapter aims to support you in transforming your microdosing journey into a catalyst for lasting positive change.

Whether you are an experienced psychonaut or just beginning to explore the world of microdosing, this chapter offers valuable insights and guidance on how to make the most of your microdosing experiences, creating a foundation for ongoing personal growth and self-discovery.

Tracking and Evaluating your Microdosing Experiences

To optimize your microdosing journey and fully understand its impact on your well-being, tracking and evaluating your experiences is essential. By monitoring your progress, you can make informed decisions about dosage adjustments, schedule changes, and the overall effectiveness of microdosing for your personal goals.

Importance of tracking and evaluating: Tracking and evaluating your microdosing experiences are crucial for several reasons:

- Identifying patterns: Monitoring your experiences can reveal patterns in how microdosing affects your mood, cognition, and overall well-being.
- Making adjustments: By evaluating your progress, you can make informed decisions about dosage, schedule, or other changes to enhance your microdosing experience.
- Assessing effectiveness: Tracking your experiences allows you to objectively assess the effectiveness of microdosing in meeting your personal goals and expectations.

Methods for tracking and evaluating: There are several methods to help you track and evaluate your microdosing experiences:

- Journaling: Keep a detailed journal of your microdosing journey, noting the dosage, timing, effects, side effects, and insights gained. Reflect on your entries periodically to identify patterns and areas for improvement.
- Mood tracking: Utilize mood tracking apps or create a simple chart to monitor changes in mood, energy, and well-being throughout the microdosing process. Analyze your mood data to evaluate the impact of microdosing on your emotional state.
- Cognitive assessments: Perform regular cognitive assessments using online tools or apps to evaluate potential changes in cognitive function, memory, or problem-solving abilities. Compare your results over time

to assess the impact of microdosing on cognitive performance.

- Goal setting and reflection: Set specific, measurable goals for your microdosing journey and regularly reflect on your progress towards these goals. Use this information to make adjustments and optimize your experience.

Using your insights for improvement: Once you have gathered data and insights from tracking and evaluating your microdosing experiences, use this information to improve your journey:

- Adjust dosage: If you notice patterns of side effects or limited benefits, consider adjusting your dosage to find the optimal amount for your needs.
- Modify schedule: If your current microdosing schedule isn't providing the desired effects or is causing unwanted side effects, experiment with alternative schedules to find a better fit.
- Integrate complementary practices: Based on your insights, explore complementary practices, such as meditation, exercise, or therapy, to enhance the benefits of microdosing.
- Revisit your goals: Regularly reevaluate your personal goals for microdosing and adjust your regimen as needed to better align with these objectives.

In conclusion, tracking and evaluating your microdosing experiences are essential for optimizing your journey and understanding the impact of microdosing on your well-being. By employing various tracking methods and using the insights gained to make informed adjustments, you can maximize the potential benefits of microdosing and better achieve your personal goals.

Integrating Insights into Daily Life

One of the primary goals of microdosing with psychedelic mushrooms is to gain insights and experiences that can be integrated into daily life, leading to personal growth and improved well-being. By consciously applying these insights to various aspects of your life, you can create lasting positive change. This section covers the importance of integrating insights, strategies for doing so, and areas of life that can benefit from the integration process.

Importance of integrating insights: Integrating insights from your microdosing experiences is vital for several reasons:

- Sustained benefits: Applying the insights and lessons learned during microdosing to daily life can help maintain and reinforce the positive effects, even after stopping the microdosing regimen.
- Personal growth: Integrating insights can lead to a deeper understanding of yourself, your values, and your life goals, fostering personal growth and development.
- Improved relationships: Insights gained during microdosing can enhance empathy, communication, and understanding, leading to more fulfilling relationships with others.

Strategies for integrating insights: To effectively integrate the insights from your microdosing journey into daily life, consider the following strategies:

- Reflect on your experiences: Regularly review your journal entries, mood tracking data, and cognitive assessments to identify patterns and insights that can be applied to daily life.
- Set actionable goals: Develop specific, measurable, and achievable goals based on the insights gained during

microdosing. Break these goals down into smaller, manageable steps to ensure progress.

- Mindfulness practices: Engage in mindfulness practices, such as meditation, breathwork, or yoga, to cultivate greater self-awareness and a deeper connection to your experiences and insights.
- Seek support: Share your insights with your support network, and discuss ways to apply these lessons to daily life. They can provide valuable feedback, encouragement, and accountability.
- Be patient and persistent: Integrating insights into daily life may take time and consistent effort. Practice patience and remain committed to the process, even when challenges arise.

Areas of life benefiting from integration: Various aspects of your life can benefit from the integration of insights gained during microdosing:

- Mental health: Apply insights related to self-awareness, emotional resilience, and coping strategies to better manage stress, anxiety, and depression.
- Creativity and productivity: Use lessons learned about problem-solving, lateral thinking, and focus to enhance your creative and professional pursuits.
- Relationships: Incorporate insights about empathy, communication, and understanding to improve your connections with friends, family, and romantic partners.
- Personal growth: Apply self-discoveries and insights to your personal development, setting goals that align with your values, passions, and life purpose.
- Spiritual development: Integrate insights about your connection to the self and the world around you into your spiritual practices, fostering a deeper sense of meaning and purpose.

In conclusion, integrating insights from your microdosing journey into daily life is essential for creating lasting positive change and personal growth. By reflecting on your experiences, setting actionable goals, and applying these insights to various aspects of your life, you can maximize the benefits of microdosing and foster a greater sense of well-being and fulfillment.

Knowing When to Stop or Take Breaks

While microdosing can offer various benefits, it is crucial to recognize when to stop or take breaks to ensure your well-being and prevent potential side effects or issues. This section covers the importance of knowing when to stop or take breaks, signs that it may be time to pause or end your microdosing journey, and suggestions for maintaining the benefits during breaks.

Importance of stopping or taking breaks: Knowing when to stop or take breaks from microdosing is essential for several reasons:

- Preventing tolerance: Regularly taking breaks can help prevent the development of tolerance to the active compounds in psychedelic mushrooms, ensuring their continued effectiveness.
- Minimizing side effects: Pausing or stopping microdosing can help mitigate potential side effects, such as increased anxiety or disturbances in sleep patterns.
- Assessing progress: Taking breaks allows you to evaluate the impact of microdosing on your life and determine whether it is still necessary or beneficial to continue.

Signs it may be time to stop or take a break: Pay attention to the following signs that may indicate it's time to pause or end your microdosing journey:

- Diminished benefits: If you find that the positive effects of microdosing are no longer as noticeable or impactful, it may be time to take a break or reevaluate your dosage and schedule.
- Increased side effects: If you experience adverse side effects, such as heightened anxiety, mood swings, or sleep disturbances, consider pausing your microdosing regimen to reassess your approach.
- Achieving personal goals: If you have reached the goals you initially set for your microdosing journey, it may be time to stop or take a break to focus on integrating the insights and benefits into your daily life.
- Personal circumstances: Changes in your personal life, such as new responsibilities or stressors, may warrant taking a break from microdosing to prioritize your well-being and stability.

Maintaining benefits during breaks: To maintain the positive effects of microdosing during breaks, consider the following strategies:

- Continue mindfulness practices: Engage in meditation, breathwork, or yoga to maintain self-awareness, stress reduction, and mental clarity during breaks.
- Foster personal growth: Continue working on personal growth and development by setting new goals, engaging in self-reflection, and applying the insights gained from microdosing.
- Maintain your support network: Stay connected with your support network to discuss your experiences, maintain accountability, and receive encouragement during breaks.
- Revisit your microdosing journal: Review your microdosing journal regularly to remind yourself of the insights and lessons learned, and consider how to apply them to your daily life.

In conclusion, knowing when to stop or take breaks from microdosing is essential for maintaining well-being and ensuring the continued effectiveness of the practice. By paying attention to signs that it may be time to pause or end your microdosing journey and employing strategies to maintain the benefits during breaks, you can optimize your overall experience and personal growth.

The Future of Microdosing and Psychedelic Medicine

As we stand on the precipice of a new era in the understanding and application of psychedelic substances, the future of microdosing and psychedelic medicine appears to be full of potential and promise. With an ever-increasing body of research, anecdotal evidence, and growing mainstream acceptance, we are witnessing a paradigm shift in the way we approach mental health, well-being, and personal growth.

In this chapter, we will delve into the future of microdosing and psychedelic medicine, exploring the current research landscape, promising applications, and the potential for mainstream adoption of these transformative practices. We will also examine the ethical considerations and challenges that may arise as the field continues to evolve and expand, touching on topics such as accessibility, regulation, and the role of traditional psychedelic use in modern therapeutic contexts.

This chapter offers a thought-provoking glimpse into the future of psychedelic medicine, inviting you to imagine the possibilities and join the conversation as we collectively forge a path towards a more integrated, compassionate, and holistic approach to healing and self-discovery.

Current Research and promising applications

The field of psychedelic research has experienced a resurgence in recent years, with an increasing number of studies investigating the potential benefits and applications of psychedelic substances, including microdosing. This section covers the current state of research, promising applications, and areas where further investigation is needed.

Current state of research: While the majority of research on psychedelic substances has focused on full doses, there is a growing interest in understanding the effects and potential benefits of microdosing. Research on microdosing is still in its early stages, but preliminary findings suggest possible benefits in several areas, such as mood enhancement, cognitive improvement, and creativity.

Promising applications: Several promising applications of microdosing have emerged from current research and anecdotal reports:

- Mental health: Studies suggest that microdosing may help alleviate symptoms of anxiety, depression, and PTSD. However, more rigorous clinical trials are needed to confirm these findings and determine the most effective microdosing protocols for specific conditions.
- Cognitive enhancement: Preliminary research and anecdotal reports indicate that microdosing may improve focus, memory, and problem-solving abilities.
- Creativity and innovation: Many users report increased creativity, open-mindedness, and divergent thinking while microdosing. Additional studies are needed to understand the full scope of these effects and how they may be utilized in various professional and artistic pursuits.
- Mindfulness and well-being: Microdosing may promote mindfulness, emotional resilience, and a deeper connection to the self and the world. Research is needed to explore these effects further and determine how they can be harnessed to improve overall well-being.

Areas for further investigation: There are several areas where more research is needed to fully understand the effects and potential benefits of microdosing:

- Long-term safety and side effects: While microdosing is generally considered safe, little is known about the potential long-term effects or risks associated with the practice. More extensive studies are needed to determine the safety and possible side effects of long-term microdosing.
- Optimal dosage and schedule: Research is needed to establish the most effective dosage and schedules for various conditions and goals, as well as to understand the relationship between individual differences and optimal microdosing protocols.
- Mechanisms of action: Understanding how microdosing affects the brain and the underlying mechanisms responsible for its benefits will help refine the practice and optimize its therapeutic potential.
- Contraindications and interactions: Further research is needed to identify potential contraindications and interactions between microdosing and other medications or medical conditions, ensuring the safety and efficacy of the practice.

In conclusion, current research on microdosing with psychedelic mushrooms is still in its infancy, but preliminary findings and anecdotal reports suggest promising applications in mental health, cognitive enhancement, creativity, and overall well-being. As the field of psychedelic research continues to expand, microdosing is likely to play an increasingly significant role in therapeutic and personal growth contexts.

The Potential for Mainstream Adoption

As research into microdosing with psychedelic mushrooms continues to grow and reveal promising results, the potential for mainstream adoption becomes more feasible. This section discusses the factors contributing to mainstream adoption, the challenges that need to be addressed, and the potential impact on society.

Factors contributing to mainstream adoption: Several factors are contributing to the increased interest in and potential for mainstream adoption of microdosing:

- Growing scientific evidence: As more studies are conducted on the safety, efficacy, and benefits of microdosing, the body of evidence supporting its use for various purposes, such as mental health and cognitive enhancement, is growing.
- Resurgence of psychedelic research: The renewed interest in psychedelic research, including the therapeutic use of substances like psilocybin, LSD, and MDMA, is helping to reduce stigma and increase awareness of the potential benefits of these substances.
- Anecdotal success stories: The increasing number of personal accounts and testimonials from individuals who have benefited from microdosing has helped to raise public interest and curiosity about the practice.
- Shifts in public opinion: As societal attitudes toward psychedelics and alternative therapies evolve, there is a growing openness to exploring the potential benefits of microdosing.

Challenges to mainstream adoption: Despite the growing interest in microdosing, several challenges must be addressed before it can become mainstream:

- Legal barriers: The legal status of psychedelic substances, including psilocybin-containing mushrooms, remains a significant barrier to widespread adoption. Efforts to decriminalize or legalize these substances in various jurisdictions may help to pave the way for more widespread acceptance and use.

- Limited research: Although research into microdosing is expanding, more rigorous, large-scale studies are needed to fully understand its potential benefits, risks, and mechanisms of action.
- Standardization and regulation: The development of standardized microdosing protocols, quality control measures, and regulatory frameworks will be crucial to ensure the safety and efficacy of microdosing as it becomes more widely adopted.
- Education and awareness: Public education efforts and accurate information dissemination will be necessary to counteract misconceptions, stigma, and misinformation surrounding microdosing and psychedelic substances in general.

Potential impact on society: If microdosing with psychedelic mushrooms becomes mainstream, several potential impacts on society may arise:

- Increased access to alternative therapies: Mainstream adoption would make microdosing more accessible to individuals seeking alternative or complementary treatments for mental health issues, cognitive enhancement, or personal growth.
- Shift in mental health care: The integration of microdosing into mental health care could lead to new treatment approaches and a broader range of options for patients.
- Enhanced creativity and innovation: The potential cognitive and creative benefits of microdosing could contribute to increased innovation and productivity in various professional and artistic fields.
- Deeper conversations about mental health and well-being: The mainstream adoption of microdosing could help to destigmatize conversations around mental

health and well-being, encouraging more open and supportive discussions.

In conclusion, the potential for mainstream adoption of microdosing with psychedelic mushrooms is growing due to increased research, anecdotal success stories, and shifts in public opinion. However, challenges such as legal barriers, limited research, and the need for standardization and regulation must be addressed before widespread adoption can occur. If these challenges are overcome, the mainstream adoption of microdosing could have a significant impact on mental health care, creativity, innovation, and societal attitudes toward well-being.

Ethical Considerations and the Future of Psychedelic Therapy

As the field of psychedelic research advances and the potential benefits of substances like psilocybin-containing mushrooms become more widely recognized, it is crucial to consider the ethical implications of these therapies. This section discusses some of the key ethical considerations, as well as the future directions of psychedelic therapy.

Ethical considerations: Several ethical concerns must be addressed when considering the use of psychedelics for therapy, including:

- Informed consent: Ensuring that individuals considering psychedelic therapy are provided with accurate, comprehensive information about the potential benefits, risks, and side effects, as well as alternative treatment options, is essential for making informed decisions about their care.
- Access and equity: As psychedelic therapies become more widely available, it is crucial to address potential barriers

to access, such as financial constraints, limited availability of treatment providers, and cultural stigma, to ensure that all individuals who could benefit have equal opportunities to access these therapies.

- Safety and harm reduction: Establishing guidelines and best practices for the safe administration of psychedelic substances, including proper dosing, screening for contraindications, and providing supportive environments, is necessary to minimize potential risks and ensure patient well-being.

- Therapist training and competency: Ensuring that therapists and other treatment providers have the necessary training, expertise, and cultural competency to effectively administer and support patients undergoing psychedelic therapy is critical to promoting positive outcomes and mitigating potential harm.

The future of psychedelic therapy: As research into psychedelics continues to grow and evolve, several potential future directions for psychedelic therapy may emerge:

- Expanded therapeutic applications: As more studies are conducted on the safety and efficacy of psychedelic substances, their therapeutic applications may expand to include a wider range of mental health conditions, as well as personal growth and well-being.

- Integration into mainstream mental health care: As the evidence supporting the benefits of psychedelic therapy grows, it may become more widely accepted and integrated into mainstream mental health care, potentially leading to new treatment paradigms and approaches.

- Personalized treatment protocols: Future research may reveal the need for personalized treatment protocols based on individual factors such as genetics, personality, and the specific mental health condition being treated.

This could lead to more targeted and effective therapeutic interventions.

- Legal and regulatory changes: As public opinion shifts and the potential benefits of psychedelics become more widely recognized, changes in legal and regulatory frameworks may follow, leading to increased access to psychedelic therapies and the potential for decriminalization or legalization of certain substances.
- Ethical guidelines and professional standards: As the field of psychedelic therapy continues to grow and mature, the development and implementation of ethical guidelines and professional standards will be essential to ensure the safety, efficacy, and integrity of the practice.

In conclusion, ethical considerations play a vital role in shaping the future of psychedelic therapy. By addressing concerns related to informed consent, access, safety, and therapist training, the field can continue to evolve responsibly and effectively. As research progresses and the potential benefits of psychedelics become more widely recognized, the future of psychedelic therapy may involve expanded therapeutic applications, integration into mainstream mental health care, personalized treatment protocols, and changes in legal and regulatory frameworks. Ultimately, a commitment to ethical practice will be essential to ensuring the success and sustainability of psychedelic therapy as it continues to grow and develop.

Frequently Asked Questions

In this Frequently Asked Questions (FAQ) section, we address some of the most common questions and concerns related to microdosing psychedelic mushrooms. By providing clear and concise answers, we aim to enhance your understanding of microdosing and dispel any misconceptions that might arise as you explore this powerful and transformative practice.

What is microdosing?

Microdosing is the practice of consuming small, sub-perceptual amounts of a psychedelic substance, such as psilocybin mushrooms, to achieve various cognitive, emotional, and physical benefits without experiencing the typical hallucinogenic effects of a full dose.

Is microdosing legal?

The legality of microdosing varies by country and region. In many places, including the United States, psilocybin mushrooms are considered illegal substances. However, there are some areas where possession and use of psychedelic mushrooms are decriminalized or regulated for therapeutic use. It's important to understand the laws and regulations in your specific location before engaging in microdosing.

How much should I microdose?

The ideal microdose varies depending on the individual and the specific type of psychedelic mushroom being used. Generally, a microdose of psilocybin mushrooms ranges from 0.1 to 0.5 grams of dried material. It's recommended to start with a lower dose and gradually adjust based on your personal experience and needs.

How often should I microdose?

A common microdosing schedule involves consuming a microdose once every three days, allowing for two days in between doses to minimize potential tolerance build-up and to fully integrate the effects of the microdose. However, individual preferences and needs may vary, and it's essential to find the schedule that works best for you.

Are there any side effects or risks associated with microdosing?

While microdosing is generally considered safe and well-tolerated, there can be potential side effects and risks, such as increased anxiety, changes in mood, or interactions with medications. It's crucial to be aware of these risks, monitor your reactions, and consult a healthcare professional if you have concerns or experience adverse effects.

Can I microdose while taking medications?

Microdosing while on medications can present potential risks, particularly with drugs that interact with serotonin, such as SSRIs or MAOIs. It's essential to consult a healthcare professional before microdosing if you are taking medications or have pre-existing health conditions.

How long does it take to notice the benefits of microdosing?

The benefits of microdosing can vary from person to person, with some individuals noticing effects within a few days, while others may require several weeks or more to experience significant changes. It's essential to be patient, maintain a consistent microdosing schedule, and track your experiences to gauge the effectiveness of your microdosing regimen.

Can I build a tolerance to microdosing?

It is possible to develop a tolerance to psilocybin when microdosing too frequently. To avoid this, it's essential to follow a responsible microdosing schedule, such as the commonly recommended "one day on, two days off" approach.

Will microdosing interfere with my daily activities?

A proper microdose should not cause significant disruptions to your daily activities. The purpose of microdosing is to experience subtle, yet noticeable, benefits without the intense effects associated with a full psychedelic dose. However, it's essential to monitor your reactions and adjust your dosage accordingly to ensure a positive and productive experience.

Can I combine microdosing with other supplements or substances?

Many individuals choose to combine microdosing with other supplements, such as Lion's Mane or Niacin, to enhance the effects or target specific outcomes. However, it's crucial to research and understand the potential interactions between substances and consult a healthcare professional if you're uncertain or have concerns.

Is microdosing addictive?

Psilocybin mushrooms are not considered to be physically addictive, and there is a low potential for psychological dependence when used responsibly. However, as with any substance, it's essential to approach microdosing with intention, mindfulness, and self-awareness to minimize any potential risks.

Can I microdose if I have a history of mental health issues?

Individuals with a history of mental health issues should approach microdosing with caution, as it may exacerbate certain conditions or interact with medications. It's crucial to consult with a healthcare professional before beginning a microdosing regimen if you have a history of mental health concerns or are currently receiving treatment.

How long should I continue microdosing?

The ideal duration of a microdosing regimen varies depending on the individual and their specific goals. Some people may choose to microdose for a few weeks or months, while others may continue for a more extended period. It's essential to regularly evaluate your experiences, track your progress, and make adjustments as needed to ensure a beneficial and safe microdosing experience.

Is it safe to drive or operate machinery while microdosing?

As microdosing involves sub-perceptual doses, it should not cause significant impairment in motor skills or cognition. However, it's essential to understand your personal reactions to microdosing and avoid engaging in potentially hazardous activities if you feel your abilities may be compromised.

Can I microdose while pregnant or breastfeeding?
The safety of microdosing during pregnancy or breastfeeding is not well understood, and there is limited research available on this topic. It's essential to prioritize the health and well-being of both the mother and child during these periods, and it is generally not recommended to microdose during pregnancy or while breastfeeding. If you're considering microdosing during these times, it's crucial to consult a healthcare professional for guidance.

Will microdosing interact with my current medications?
Microdosing may interact with certain medications, particularly those that affect the serotonin system, such as selective serotonin reuptake inhibitors (SSRIs) or monoamine oxidase inhibitors (MAOIs). It's important to consult with a healthcare professional before beginning a microdosing regimen if you're currently taking medications or have concerns about potential interactions.

How can I find a community or support network for microdosing?
Connecting with like-minded individuals or support networks can be a valuable aspect of the microdosing journey. Online forums, social media groups, and local meet-ups focused on psychedelic exploration or microdosing may be good places to start. Remember to be cautious about sharing personal information and experiences, especially given the legal status of psychedelic substances in some areas.

What should I do if I have a negative experience while microdosing?
If you encounter a challenging experience while microdosing, it's essential to remain calm and remind yourself that the effects are temporary. Taking slow, deep breaths and engaging in grounding

techniques, such as meditation or spending time in nature, can help you regain a sense of balance. It's also helpful to have a support network or a trusted individual who can provide guidance and reassurance during difficult moments. Reflect on your experience, consider adjusting your dosage or schedule, and consult a professional if necessary.

Can I travel with psychedelic mushrooms or microdose while abroad?

Traveling with psychedelic substances, including psilocybin mushrooms, can be risky due to varying laws and regulations in different countries. It's crucial to be aware of and comply with the laws and regulations in the countries you plan to visit. Additionally, it's essential to consider the potential risks and challenges of microdosing in an unfamiliar environment and prioritize your safety and well-being.

If you have further questions or concerns about microdosing psychedelic mushrooms, we encourage you to explore the rest of the chapters in this book, where we delve deeper into various aspects of microdosing, its potential benefits, and practical considerations.

Personal Accounts

These stories provide unique perspectives on the potential benefits and challenges of microdosing, offering valuable insights to those interested in exploring this practice for themselves.

Alice's Creative Reawakening: Alice, a graphic designer, struggled with creative burnout and a lack of inspiration in her work. After starting a microdosing regimen, she found herself more open to new ideas and artistic styles. Her creativity flourished, and she was able to complete several new projects that she had previously been struggling with.

Ben's Journey Through Social Anxiety: Ben had always struggled with social anxiety, which made it difficult for him to make friends and enjoy social events. After he began microdosing, he noticed a significant decrease in his anxiety levels and a newfound confidence in social situations. Over time, he formed deeper connections with others and started enjoying social events more.

Carla's Path to Emotional Healing: Carla, a survivor of childhood trauma, had tried various therapies without success. When she started microdosing, she experienced a breakthrough in her emotional healing process. The practice allowed her to confront and work through her past traumas, leading to a sense of inner peace and emotional resilience.

David's Athletic Performance: David, an amateur runner, turned to microdosing to improve his athletic performance. He found that it not only boosted his physical stamina but also improved his mental focus during long runs. As a result, he was able to achieve personal bests in several races and enjoyed his training sessions more.

Eva's Spiritual Awakening: Eva, a long-time spiritual seeker, decided to try microdosing as part of her meditation practice. She discovered that it helped her achieve a deeper state of mindfulness and self-awareness. Microdosing also facilitated profound insights and a stronger connection to her inner self and the world around her.

Frank's Improved Sleep: Frank had struggled with insomnia for years, which affected his overall well-being and productivity. After starting a microdosing regimen, he found that his sleep patterns improved significantly, leading to more restorative rest and a better quality of life.

Grace's Enhanced Problem-Solving: Grace, a software engineer, faced challenges in her work that required innovative solutions. She started microdosing and noticed her ability to think laterally and approach problems from new angles had improved. Consequently, she became a more effective problem solver and contributed innovative ideas to her team.

Henry's Battle with Depression: Henry had been living with depression for many years, finding little relief from traditional medications. He decided to try microdosing as a last resort. To his surprise, his mood improved, and his depressive episodes became less frequent and less severe. Microdosing offered him a new sense of hope and control over his mental health.

Isabella's Enhanced Mindfulness Practice: As a yoga teacher and mindfulness practitioner, Isabella was always looking for ways to deepen her practice. When she started microdosing, she found that it helped her become more present, aware, and connected to her body during her practice. Her students also noticed the improvements in her teaching style and her ability to create a more mindful environment.

Jack's Journey with PTSD: Jack, a military veteran, struggled with post-traumatic stress disorder (PTSD) after returning from combat. Traditional therapies had limited success in helping him manage his symptoms. After starting a microdosing regimen, Jack noticed a significant reduction in his anxiety, flashbacks, and overall distress. Microdosing provided him with a valuable tool for coping with his PTSD.

Karen's Improved Work-Life Balance: Karen, a busy executive, found it challenging to balance her demanding career with her personal life. She often felt stressed, overwhelmed, and burned out. After incorporating microdosing into her routine, she experienced increased focus, energy, and mental clarity, allowing her to be more efficient at work and have more time and energy for her personal life.

Liam's Overcoming Creative Block: Liam, a professional painter, found himself in the midst of a creative block, struggling to produce new work. After incorporating microdosing into his routine, he discovered renewed inspiration, creativity, and a fresh perspective on his art. His productivity and artistic expression flourished, leading to several successful exhibitions.

Mia's Enhanced Athletic Performance: As a dedicated amateur runner, Mia sought ways to improve her performance and endurance. When she began microdosing, she experienced heightened mental stamina and a stronger connection between her mind and body, enabling her to push past her limits and achieve personal bests.

Noah's Improved Relationships: Noah had difficulty connecting with others and maintaining healthy relationships, due in part to his social anxiety. After starting a microdosing regimen, he noticed increased empathy, emotional openness, and self-confidence, which transformed his interactions with friends and family and strengthened his relationships.

Olivia's Spiritual Growth: Olivia, a spiritual seeker, was always looking for ways to deepen her connection with the divine. When she began microdosing, she found that her meditation and contemplative practices became more profound and transformative, fostering a more profound sense of unity and interconnectedness with the world around her.

Peter's Enhanced Memory and Learning: Peter, a college student, struggled with retaining information and staying focused during long study sessions. After starting microdosing, he noticed improved memory recall, concentration, and ability to absorb new information. As a result, his academic performance improved, and he found learning more enjoyable and rewarding.

These personal accounts demonstrate the diverse ways in which microdosing can positively impact individuals' lives. Each person's experience is unique, and it's important to approach microdosing with an open mind and a willingness to learn and grow.

Conclusion

As we reach the conclusion of this enlightening journey through the world of microdosing, it is essential to pause and reflect on the wealth of information, insights, and personal stories we have explored. This transformative practice has the potential to unlock new dimensions of creativity, cognitive enhancement, emotional wellbeing, and spiritual growth, offering a promising alternative to traditional pharmaceuticals and treatment methods.

In this final chapter, we will take a step back to appreciate the transformative power of microdosing, while emphasizing the importance of responsible and intentional use, and envisioning a future where psychedelic wellness is seamlessly integrated into our daily lives.

Reflecting on the Transformative Power of Microdosing

As we consider the research, anecdotal reports, and ethical implications of microdosing with psychedelic mushrooms, it becomes clear that microdosing has the potential to be a transformative practice for many individuals. This section reflects on the transformative power of microdosing and its potential impact on personal growth, mental health, and overall well-being.

Personal growth and self-exploration: Microdosing can offer a unique opportunity for personal growth and self-exploration, as it may facilitate introspection, enhance self-awareness, and promote a deeper connection to the self and the world. By fostering these qualities, microdosing can help individuals better understand their thoughts, emotions, and behaviors, ultimately enabling them to make more informed choices and engage in more fulfilling, authentic lives.

Mental health and emotional resilience: The potential of microdosing to alleviate symptoms of anxiety, depression, and stress highlights its transformative power in the realm of mental health. By supporting emotional resilience, boosting mood, and fostering a sense of well-being, microdosing can provide individuals with the tools to navigate life's challenges more effectively and cultivate a greater sense of overall happiness.

Cognitive enhancement and creativity: The cognitive benefits of microdosing, such as improved focus, memory, and problem-solving abilities, can contribute to personal and professional success, enabling individuals to unlock their full potential. Furthermore, the reported enhancement of creativity and divergent thinking can lead to innovative breakthroughs and novel approaches to both artistic and professional pursuits, transforming the way individuals approach their work and passions.

Mindfulness and spiritual growth: Microdosing can also support mindfulness and spiritual growth, fostering a greater sense of presence and connection to the present moment. As individuals become more mindful and in tune with their inner selves, they may find it easier to cultivate gratitude, compassion, and a deeper sense of meaning and purpose in their lives.

Societal impact: On a broader scale, the transformative power of microdosing could contribute to a shift in societal attitudes towards mental health, well-being, and personal growth. As more people experience the benefits of microdosing and share their stories, conversations around mental health and self-improvement may become more open and destigmatized, paving the way for a more compassionate and supportive society.

In conclusion, the transformative power of microdosing with psychedelic mushrooms lies in its potential to facilitate personal growth, support mental health, enhance cognitive abilities, and promote mindfulness and spiritual development. As research continues to uncover the potential benefits and applications of microdosing, it may become an increasingly valuable tool for individuals seeking to improve their lives, foster a deeper connection to themselves and others, and contribute to a more compassionate and understanding society.

Encouraging Responsible and Intentional Use

As interest in microdosing with psychedelic mushrooms continues to grow, it is essential to promote responsible and intentional use to ensure the safety and well-being of those who choose to explore this practice. This section highlights the importance of approaching microdosing with a sense of responsibility, intention, and mindfulness.

Education and accurate information: The foundation of responsible and intentional microdosing begins with educating oneself and seeking accurate information about the potential benefits, risks, and best practices. By understanding the science, mechanisms, and effects of microdosing, individuals can make informed decisions about their own use and minimize potential risks.

Mindful intention-setting: Approaching microdosing with a clear and specific intention can help individuals optimize their experience and derive the most significant benefits. Intention-setting involves reflecting on one's goals, motivations, and desired outcomes, which might include personal growth, mental health improvement, or enhanced creativity. By setting intentions, individuals can cultivate a greater sense of purpose and direction throughout their microdosing journey.

Proper dosing and scheduling: Responsible microdosing involves adhering to appropriate dosing and scheduling guidelines to minimize potential risks and ensure optimal results. This includes accurately measuring doses, following recommended microdosing schedules, and adjusting as needed based on personal tolerance and individual responses.

Self-monitoring and evaluation: Regular self-monitoring and evaluation are crucial aspects of responsible microdosing. By tracking their experiences, individuals can gain valuable insights into how microdosing is affecting them, identify potential side effects or concerns, and make adjustments as needed to optimize their experience.

Legal considerations and safety: It is essential to be aware of and respect the legal status of psychedelic substances in one's jurisdiction, as well as to prioritize safety by considering potential contraindications, precautions, and harm reduction strategies. This includes screening for medical or psychological conditions that may increase risk, creating a supportive and comfortable environment, and having a trusted support network available if needed.

Integration of insights and personal growth: Responsible microdosing involves not only the act of taking a substance but also the integration of insights and personal growth derived from the experience. This includes engaging in self-reflection, journaling, or discussing experiences with a support network or therapist to gain a deeper understanding of the changes and growth occurring during the microdosing journey.

Ethical sourcing and sustainability: Considering the ethical implications of sourcing psychedelic mushrooms is another important aspect of responsible use. This includes researching the origins of the mushrooms, ensuring they are obtained from sustainable and ethical sources, and considering the ecological impact of their production and consumption.

By promoting responsible and intentional use, individuals can approach microdosing with psychedelic mushrooms in a manner that supports their well-being, personal growth, and overall safety. By prioritizing education, intention-setting, proper dosing, self-monitoring, legal considerations, integration, and ethical sourcing, individuals can embark on their microdosing journey with mindfulness, care, and a deep sense of purpose.

Envisioning a Future of Integrated Psychedelic Wellness

As our understanding of the potential benefits of microdosing with psychedelic mushrooms and other psychedelic substances continues to evolve, it is worth considering a future where these practices are integrated into a broader framework of mental health and personal well-being. This section envisions a future of integrated psychedelic wellness, in which responsible and intentional use of psychedelic substances becomes a valuable component of holistic health and personal growth.

Accessible and destigmatized psychedelic therapies: In this envisioned future, psychedelic therapies, including microdosing, would become more widely accessible and destigmatized, with mental health professionals and treatment centers incorporating these practices into their offerings. Individuals seeking support for mental health challenges or personal growth would have access to a range of psychedelic-assisted therapies, tailored to their unique needs and preferences.

Integration with conventional therapies: Psychedelic wellness practices would be integrated with conventional therapies, such as cognitive-behavioral therapy, mindfulness-based practices, and other evidence-based approaches. This would create a more comprehensive and holistic approach to mental health care, allowing individuals to draw from a variety of therapeutic modalities to support their well-being and personal growth.

Personalized wellness plans: Integrated psychedelic wellness would involve personalized wellness plans that take into account individual factors, such as genetics, personal history, and mental health needs. This tailored approach would ensure that each person receives the most appropriate and effective combination of therapies, including microdosing, to support their unique journey toward mental and emotional well-being.

Community-based support networks: As psychedelic practices become more widely accepted and integrated into mental health care, community-based support networks would emerge to help individuals navigate their experiences and integrate their insights. These networks may include support groups, integration circles, and workshops, providing safe spaces for individuals to share, learn, and grow together.

Ongoing research and development: In a future of integrated psychedelic wellness, ongoing research and development would continue to deepen our understanding of the potential benefits, risks, and mechanisms of microdosing and other psychedelic practices. This research would inform the development of best practices, guidelines, and innovative therapeutic approaches, ensuring that individuals have access to the most effective and evidence-based treatments.

Ethical and sustainable practices: In this envisioned future, the ethical and sustainable sourcing of psychedelic substances, such as mushrooms, would be prioritized, ensuring that these practices have minimal ecological impact and support equitable access. Moreover, the development of professional standards and ethical guidelines would help safeguard the integrity and safety of psychedelic-assisted therapies.

By integrating psychedelic wellness practices into a broader framework of mental health care and personal well-being, we can envision a future where the responsible and intentional use of substances like psychedelic mushrooms becomes a valuable component of holistic health and personal growth. In this future, individuals would have access to a range of evidence-based therapies, personalized wellness plans, and supportive community networks, enabling them to embark on transformative journeys toward mental, emotional, and spiritual well-being.

Resources and Further Reading

Books

1. Fadiman, J. (2011). The Psychedelic Explorer's Guide: Safe, Therapeutic, and Sacred Journeys. Park Street Press.
2. Pollan, M. (2018). How to Change Your Mind: What the New Science of Psychedelics Teaches Us About Consciousness, Dying, Addiction, Depression, and Transcendence. Penguin Press.
3. Stamets, P. (1996). Psilocybin Mushrooms of the World: An Identification Guide. Ten Speed Press.
4. Hartogsohn, I. (2020). American Trip: Set, Setting, and the Psychedelic Experience in the Twentieth Century. MIT Press.
5. Waldman, A. (2017). A Really Good Day: How Microdosing Made a Mega Difference in My Mood, My Marriage, and My Life. Alfred A. Knopf.
6. Letcher, A. (2007). Shroom: A Cultural History of the Magic Mushroom. Faber & Faber.
7. Shroder, T. (2014). Acid Test: LSD, Ecstasy, and the Power to Heal. Blue Rider Press.
8. Huxley, A. (1954). The Doors of Perception and Heaven and Hell. Harper & Brothers.
9. Thorne, B. (2021). Microdosing Psychedelics: A Practical Guide to Upgrade Your Life. Independently published.
10. Smith, R. E. (2020). Psychedelic Medicine: The Healing Powers of LSD, MDMA, Psilocybin, and Ayahuasca. Watkins Media.

Articles

1. Carhart-Harris, R. L., & Goodwin, G. M. (2017). The Therapeutic Potential of Psychedelic Drugs: Past, Present, and Future. Neuropsychopharmacology.
2. Fadiman, J., & Korb, S. (2019). Might microdosing psychedelics be safe and beneficial? An initial exploration. Journal of Psychoactive Drugs, 51(2), 118-122.
3. Kuypers, K. P. C., Ng, L., Erritzoe, D., Knudsen, G. M., Nichols, C. D., Nichols, D. E., Pani, L., Soula, A., & Nutt, D. (2019). Microdosing psychedelics: More questions than answers? An overview and suggestions for future research. Journal of Psychopharmacology, 33(9), 1039-1057.
4. Johnstad, P. G. (2018). Powerful substances in tiny amounts: An interview study of psychedelic microdosing. Nordic Studies on Alcohol and Drugs, 35(1), 39-51.
5. Polito, V., & Stevenson, R. J. (2019). A systematic study of microdosing psychedelics. PLoS ONE, 14(2), e0211023.
6. Anderson, T., Petranker, R., Christopher, A., Rosenbaum, D., Weissman, C., Dinh-Williams, L., Hui, K., Hapke, E., & Farb, N. (2019). Psychedelic microdosing benefits and challenges: An empirical codebook. Harm Reduction Journal, 16(1), 43.
7. Cameron, L. P., & Olson, D. E. (2018). Dark classics in chemical neuroscience: Psilocybin. ACS Chemical Neuroscience, 9(10), 2438-2447.

Movies and Documentaries

1. Fantastic Fungi (2019). Directed by Louie Schwartzberg. Moving Art Studio.
2. DMT: The Spirit Molecule (2010). Directed by Mitch Schultz. Spectral Alchemy, Synthetic Pictures.

3. Dosed (2019) - Directed by Tyler Chandler, this documentary follows the journey of an opioid addict who turns to the healing powers of psychedelic substances, including microdosing, as a means to overcome her addiction.

4. The Mind Explained: Psychedelics (2019) - This episode from the Netflix series "The Mind, Explained" delves into the science and history of psychedelics, including microdosing, and features interviews with experts and enthusiasts.

5. The Psychedelic Renaissance (2021) - Directed by Guy Harrington, this documentary explores the potential of psychedelic substances for mental health treatment and wellness, including the practice of microdosing.

6. The Spirit Molecule (2010) - This documentary, based on the book by Dr. Rick Strassman, discusses the powerful psychedelic substance DMT and its potential effects on human consciousness. Though not specifically focused on microdosing, it offers valuable insights into the world of psychedelics.

7. Fantastic Fungi (2019) - Directed by Louie Schwartzberg, this documentary dives deep into the world of fungi, exploring their importance to our ecosystem and their potential for healing, including the use of psilocybin mushrooms for microdosing.

8. Neurons to Nirvana (2013) - This documentary by Oliver Hockenhull explores the history, science, and potential benefits of psychedelic substances, including the practice of microdosing for personal growth and cognitive enhancement.

Podcasts

1. The Psychedelic Salon: Hosted by Lorenzo Hagerty, The Psychedelic Salon is a podcast that features interviews,

lectures, and talks with some of the most prominent figures in the field of psychedelics.

2. The Third Wave Podcast: Hosted by Paul Austin, The Third Wave Podcast focuses on the responsible use of psychedelics for personal growth and transformation.

3. Adventures Through The Mind - Hosted by James W. Jesso, this podcast explores various topics related to psychedelics, consciousness, and personal development, often featuring interviews with experts and researchers.

4. The Psychedelic Experience - Hosted by Joe Moore, this podcast offers a variety of discussions and interviews related to the world of psychedelics, including microdosing, integration, and the latest research findings.

5. The Entheogenic Evolution - Hosted by Martin W. Ball, this podcast delves into the world of entheogens and their potential for healing, transformation, and personal growth, with a focus on microdosing and other responsible uses of psychedelics.

6. The DoseNation Podcast - This podcast covers a wide range of topics related to psychedelics, drug policy, and the science of altered states, often featuring interviews with experts and thought leaders in the field.

7. The MAPS (Multidisciplinary Association for Psychedelic Studies) Podcast - Hosted by Zach Leary, this podcast provides in-depth interviews with researchers, scientists, and advocates working on the cutting edge of psychedelic research and policy reform.

8. The Tim Ferriss Show - Though not exclusively focused on psychedelics, host Tim Ferriss often discusses the topic of microdosing and features interviews with leading experts in the field, such as Dr. James Fadiman and Paul Stamets.

Websites and Organizations

1. The Beckley Foundation: A non-profit organization that focuses on groundbreaking psychedelic research and

promoting evidence-based drug policy reform. Website: https://www.beckleyfoundation.org/

2. Multidisciplinary Association for Psychedelic Studies (MAPS): A non-profit research and educational organization that develops medical, legal, and cultural contexts for people to benefit from the careful uses of psychedelics. Website: https://maps.org/

3. The Third Wave (https://thethirdwave.co/) - The Third Wave is an online resource that provides information, education, and resources on the responsible use of psychedelics, including comprehensive guides on microdosing and its benefits.

4. The Psychedelic Science (https://www.psychedelicscience.org/) - This website is a hub for the latest research, news, and events related to psychedelic science, including studies and resources on microdosing.

5. Shroomery (https://www.shroomery.org/) - Shroomery is an online community dedicated to the discussion and cultivation of psychedelic mushrooms, including resources and forums on microdosing.

6. Erowid (https://www.erowid.org/) - Erowid is a comprehensive online resource that provides information on psychoactive substances, including psychedelics and microdosing, with an extensive library of articles, research, and personal experiences.

7. The DMT Nexus (https://www.dmt-nexus.me/) - The DMT Nexus is an online community focused on the exploration and discussion of DMT, ayahuasca, and other psychedelics, with resources and forums related to microdosing and personal experiences.

8. The Psychedelic Experience (https://www.psychedelicexperience.net/) - This website offers a platform for users to share and explore personal experiences with psychedelics, including microdosing, as

well as resources and information on safe and responsible use.

9. The Psychedelic Society (https://psychedelicsociety.org.uk/) - The Psychedelic Society is an organization that advocates for the responsible use of psychedelics and provides events, workshops, and resources related to microdosing and personal growth.

10. Chacruna Institute (https://chacruna.net/) - The Chacruna Institute is a non-profit organization that promotes plant medicines and indigenous knowledge, including research, education, and resources on microdosing and responsible use of psychedelics.

References

1. Anderson, T., Petranker, R., Christopher, A., Rosenbaum, D., Weissman, C., Dinh-Williams, L.-A., ... Hui, K. (2021). Psychedelic microdosing benefits and challenges: An empirical codebook. Harm Reduction Journal, 18(1), 1–16. https://doi.org/10.1186/s12954-020-00408-6

2. Carhart-Harris, R. L., Bolstridge, M., Rucker, J., Day, C. M., Erritzoe, D., Kaelen, M., ... & Taylor, D. (2016). Psilocybin with psychological support for treatment-resistant depression: An open-label feasibility study. The Lancet Psychiatry, 3(7), 619-627. https://doi.org/10.1016/S2215-0366(16)30065-7

3. Davis, A. K., Barrett, F. S., May, D. G., Cosimano, M. P., Sepeda, N. D., Johnson, M. W., ... & Griffiths, R. R. (2021). Effects of psilocybin-assisted therapy on major depressive disorder: A randomized clinical trial. JAMA Psychiatry, 78(5), 481-489. https://doi.org/10.1001/jamapsychiatry.2021.0158

4. Fadiman, J., & Korb, S. (2019). Might microdosing psychedelics be safe and beneficial? An initial exploration. Journal of Psychoactive Drugs, 51(2), 118-122. https://doi.org/10.1080/02791072.2019.1593561

5. Fuentes, J. J., Fonseca, F., Elices, M., Farré, M., & Torrens, M. (2020). Therapeutic use of LSD in psychiatry: A systematic review of randomized-controlled clinical trials. Frontiers in Psychiatry, 10, 943. https://doi.org/10.3389/fpsyt.2019.00943

6. Griffiths, R. R., Johnson, M. W., Carducci, M. A., Umbricht, A., Richards, W. A., Richards, B. D., ... & Klinedinst, M. A. (2016). Psilocybin produces substantial and sustained decreases in depression and anxiety in patients with life-threatening cancer: A randomized double-blind trial. Journal of Psychopharmacology,

30(12), 1181-1197. https://doi.org/10.1177/0269881116675513

7. Haijen, E. C., Kaelen, M., Roseman, L., Timmermann, C., Kettner, H., Russ, S., ... & Carhart-Harris, R. L. (2018). Predicting responses to psychedelics: A prospective study. Frontiers in Pharmacology, 9, 897. https://doi.org/10.3389/fphar.2018.00897

8. Hutten, N. R., Mason, N. L., Dolder, P. C., & Kuypers, K. P. (2019). Motives and side-effects of microdosing with psychedelics among users. International Journal of Neuropsychopharmacology, 22(7), 426-434. https://doi.org/10.1093/ijnp/pyz029

9. Johnson, M. W., Griffiths, R. R., Hendricks, P. S., & Henningfield, J. E. (2018). The abuse potential of medical psilocybin according to the 8 factors of the Controlled Substances Act. Neuropharmacology, 142, 143-166. https://doi.org/10.1016/j.neuropharm.2018.05.012

10. Johnstad, P. G. (2018). Powerful substances in tiny amounts: An interview study of psychedelic microdosing. Nordic Studies on Alcohol and Drugs, 35(1), 39-51. https://doi.org/10.1177/1455072517753339

11. Krediet, E., Bostoen, T., Breeksema, J., van Schagen, A., Passie, T., & Vermetten, E. (2020). Reviewing the potential of psychedelics for the treatment of PTSD. International Journal of Neuropsychopharmacology, 23(6), 385-400. https://doi.org/10.1093/ijnp/pyaa018

12. Lyons, T., & Carhart-Harris, R. L. (2018). Increased nature relatedness and decreased authoritarian political views after psilocybin for treatment-resistant depression. Journal of Psychopharmacology, 32(7), 811-819. https://doi.org/10.1177/0269881117748902

13. Mithoefer, M. C., Wagner, M. T., Mithoefer, A. T., Jerome, L., & Doblin, R. (2011). The safety and efficacy of ±3,4-methylenedioxymethamphetamine-assisted psychotherapy in subjects with chronic, treatment-resistant posttraumatic stress disorder: The

first randomized controlled pilot study. Journal of Psychopharmacology, 25(4), 439-452. https://doi.org/10.1177/0269881110378371

14. Polito, V., & Stevenson, R. J. (2019). A systematic study of microdosing psychedelics. PLOS ONE, 14(2), e0211023. https://doi.org/10.1371/journal.pone.0211023

15. Prochazkova, L., Lippelt, D. P., Colzato, L. S., Kuchar, M., Sjoerds, Z., & Hommel, B. (2018). Exploring the effect of microdosing psychedelics on creativity in an open-label natural setting. Psychopharmacology, 235(11), 3401-3413. https://doi.org/10.1007/s00213-018-5049-7

16. Soler, J., Elices, M., Dominguez-Clavé, E., Pascual, J. C., Feilding, A., Navarro-Gil, M., ... & Riba, J. (2018). Four weekly ayahuasca sessions lead to increases in "acceptance" capacities: A comparison study with a standard 8-week mindfulness training program. Frontiers in Pharmacology, 9, 224. https://doi.org/10.3389/fphar.2018.00224

17. Watts, R., Day, C., Krzanowski, J., Nutt, D., & Carhart-Harris, R. (2017). Patients' accounts of increased "connectedness" and "acceptance" after psilocybin for treatment-resistant depression. Journal of Humanistic Psychology, 57(5), 520-564. https://doi.org/10.1177/0022167817709585

18. Yanakieva, S., Polychroni, N., Family, N., Williams, L. T. J., Luke, D. P., & Terhune, D. B. (2019). The effects of microdose LSD on time perception: A randomised, double-blind, placebo-controlled trial. Psychopharmacology, 236(4), 1159-1170. https://doi.org/10.1007/s00213-018-5119-x

19. Zeifman, R. J., & Palhano-Fontes, F. (2021). The dark side of the light: Exploring the potential negative consequences of psychedelic use. Journal of Psychedelic Studies, 5(1), 1-11. https://doi.org/10.1556/2054.2020.00192

THANKS FOR READING

Thank you for delving into "Microdosing Magic." We hope it has illuminated new perspectives on the use of psychedelic mushrooms for personal and spiritual growth.

To further personalize your journey, we invite you to Visit trueeira.com/test and discover your Microdose Personality. This unique test offers transformative insights, including a Free Personalized Microdosing Protocol tailored to your individual personality traits.

Your experiences and feedback are invaluable. Please leave a review to help guide others and enrich our community's knowledge.

Join us at True Eira as we continue to explore and embrace the journey towards self-discovery and holistic well-being.

Visit

trueeira.com/test

Find Your Microdose Personality

TRUE
EIRA

OUR MISSION

At True Eira, our mission is to guide individuals on their path to self-discovery, healing, and growth through the practice of microdosing. We provide comprehensive resources that marry ancient wisdom with modern scientific insights. Our focus is on fostering a community that values knowledge, compassion, and responsible exploration in pursuit of personal transformation. We honor traditional practices while embracing scientific advancements, creating a nurturing environment that supports individual development and contributes to the broader flourishing of humanity.

TRUE EIRA ORIGINS

True Eira emerged from Travis Eric's profound experiences with entheogens and his deep understanding of their transformative power for personal growth and healing. His journey included not just exploration but also the cultivation of mushrooms, leading him to witness firsthand how profoundly transformative microdosing can be.

Motivated by these experiences, True Eira evolved into a comprehensive platform focused on well-being and self-discovery. It has become a hub where ancient wisdom is seamlessly integrated with modern practices, offering tools and a supportive community for those embarking on their transformative journey. This platform represents a fusion of Travis's personal insights and a broader mission to guide others in unveiling their intrinsic power, aligning ancient teachings with the challenges of contemporary life.

THE ESSENCE OF TRUE EIRA

The name "True Eira" holds deep significance, inspired by Eir (or Eira), the Norse goddess of healing. In Norse mythology, Eira is known for her wisdom and expertise in healing and medicine, often associated with physical and spiritual well-being. By invoking the essence of Eira, we aim to embody her healing spirit and create a space that facilitates growth, self-discovery, and personal transformation.

The term "True" in our name signifies our commitment to authenticity and integrity in exploring the vast potential of human growth and self-discovery. We strive to provide reliable, research-based information and resources while honoring the ancient traditions that have long recognized the healing powers of various practices, including using entheogens.

Combining Eira's healing essence with our dedication to authenticity, the name "True Eira" represents our mission to empower individuals on their journey towards self-discovery, healing, and personal growth through a holistic approach, encompassing ancient and modern wisdom practices.

TRUE
EIRA

Customers Who Bought This Book Also Bought

Healing Trauma with Magic Mushrooms: A Comprehensive Guide to Microdosing and Macrodosing Psilocybin for PTSD

The Athlete's Trip: Unleashing the Potential of Magic Mushrooms for Athletic Performance

Visit

trueeira.com/test

Find Your Microdose Personality

TRUE
EIRA